Testosterone Replacement Therapy

How to Boost Testosterone Levels

(Best Natural Testosterone Booster Guide for Testosterone)

Sherman Bellanger

Published By **Bengion Cosalas**

Sherman Bellanger

Testosterone Replacement Therapy: How to Boost Testosterone Levels (Best Natural Testosterone Booster Guide for Testosterone)

ISBN   978-1-998038-63-3

No part of this guidebook shall be reproduced in any form without permission in writing from the publisher except in the case of brief quotations embodied in critical articles or reviews.

Legal & Disclaimer

Upon using the information contained in this book, you agree to hold harmless the Author from and against any damages, costs, and expenses, including any legal fees potentially resulting from the application of any of the information provided by this guide. This disclaimer applies to any damages or injury caused by the use and application, whether directly or indirectly, of any advice or information presented, whether for breach of contract, tort, negligence, personal injury, criminal intent, or under any other cause of action.

You agree to accept all risks of using the information presented inside this book. You need to consult a professional medical practitioner in order to ensure you are both able and healthy enough to participate in this program.

Table Of Contents

Chapter 1: Shoulder trap shrugs are around 40 to 50kg

And then triceps pull them and then lower.

I'm not sure if I invested a huge amount of effort in this particular gym to for a wank. But it was the most enjoyable thing that I could come up with. It's like having a short one before going into bed, just to drift out of bed with any anticipation...just hit it and pray that you don't spill anything on the walls that will be visible the world in a way that will never erase.

It's as if it's another low moment today I'm not sure, but it's yet another low moment today.

However, as I'm on medications on hand and I'm on the verge of getting them, I'm hoping I'll be in a position to overcome it and make some progress. find out what you must do in the gym to improve. This is not about snatching a slow ape sister for a step up, and maybe some financial gain in the gym that is similar to being in a prison. But, I'm talking about becoming frikkin massive and gaining some significant N000bies in the process You boner brained, dEEgeneralYT reprobaitzzzz.

It's the middle of the afternoon.

I turned the blinds to the side. I was smoking an Camel lighter cigarette in my room, and gazing through the windows at the endless rain. If my Landlady is aware of my smoking outside, she'll slap me in the room as if I were a tiny kid.

Really, I'm not smoking here at all, simply creating a little ambience. The rain is falling h.a.r.d. the mist is rising off the tarmac, the cold is biting through the windows and I just wanna close the curtains and read my latest Japanese manga books by the light of a candle...but I gotta write this frikkin novel for   you   on...

..how.....too.......much......information.......to .... BECOME THE .... KRAKEN!

I've got two litres of milk inside my purse. This isn't a calf acting as a human being and certainly not half Australian or nursing an entire litter of puppies that was abandoned by my sluggish sister...this is intended for HUMAN use only.

The weight is too much in my bag that is already burdened due to all the Christmas gifts I've put from my bag since I think of myself as that fat Santa Claus sunk in milk bowls. I've had 3 Liters of water this morning, along with massive protein and mass scoops and I'm still required to drink four more Liters of water today. I'm on 6 daily litres! I'm an exceptional Christmas snow flake. One of one trillion billion of Squillions.

I get fourteen litres of milk each day as there's not enough room in the fridge for anything more than the amount I need. I'm not having any bread-based breakfast sandwiches right now because I'm not having enough appetite to eat it at the moment. I am down to seven Liters. Wow! It's not like I'm on 6 litres of milk every day and muttering about schn00dle-n00dlesand I'm on 7 FRIKKIN LITRES every FRIKKIN every day! !

I did it yesterday...just have to test how I do each day. In the end, I'll be an enormous raging mass muscles, and a true frEAk from the natural world.

While squinting at the blinds and flicking my cigarette into the ashtray, I am wondering about it. My God, I'm turning into a fat mofo. Evidently, the majority of the weight I've gained is weight gain. If I continue to progress with this pace, I'll in the near future be extremely obese around my abdomen that is great for Santa however it could be difficult to get rid of without cutting (cutting calories back below the your daily intake to shed weight) as well as losing muscle and weight. I'd rather remain on a continuous weight loss cycle, or even a slow increase in size if I'm interpreting the term properly. I was reading about the GOMAD (gallon of milk daily that is exactly what I am doing) and it seems to be similar to critiques I've heard previously.

The GOMAD program is designed for those who are having a lot of trouble getting weight. I am not one of them. I am able to gain weight very easily. for someone like me, the process of getting weight loss is as simple as breathing.

Then I've taken the decision to go with semi-skimmed milk. It is a good idea to cut back on the fat. In the following Korean nutritional info, it is stated that it contains 16% fat content in the milk. It was a bit difficult to find it however 'JiBang' is a reference to fat.

The problem is that it doesn't appear to make sense. As according to the Dairy

Council of California says Whole milk contains 3.5 percent milk fat ....' only 3.5 percent fat? What could be the reason for it being that little? !!!??? The 16% figure on the Korean report must be referring to something else, for instance the suggested daily intake because it does not seem to make sense.

So, am planning take a break from my 7 daily litres of BITCHIN. Keep it at 6 freakin' liters right now. It's back to 4800 calories after that. And, next time I order milk I might order semi skimmed. I'll keep it for review before moving back to 6 litres right now.

Recently went to the bathroom for a poop and I was thinking that it's not so bad at all however, it's not an excellent results. There are six Liters of milk within the stomach. I'm not 100% sure however there is plenty of fat as well.

This isn't satisfactory, therefore we must take action.

There are a lot of concerns about whether it is all milk, or could it be the huge amount of calories and turning me into Santa? It seems like the most effective factor to consider is to ensure that the calories are high and decrease the fat proportion however, if you do that I'm assuming that the low fat milk is about 350 calories about 350 calories per carton. This lowers daily calories enough that I'd need to consume ten large Bitchin' Liquires.

Bodybuilding is a complex subject enough for me to understand when I'm just drinking milk and a little powder. What are the other common individuals cope with eating actual foods? You must be at least a little autism-prone, anti-Australian maths head genius in order to figure out how to make the right calories, I'd think. Sick sonuvbitches. Don't ignore the need to make an effort to achieve 1-1.5 pounds of protein for each pounds of body weight, which is just 15% fat as well as 400 grams of carbohydrates at least.

And then you'll have the medication. The best part is that you can take them. One of the easiest ways to get rid of it is to see if you can get HGH recommended at around 2-4 international units. HGH can be obtained by people older than 30 certainly. You can ask your GP If you're located in the UK. If you're somewhere other than the UK, consult your physician or phone one of the anti-aging clinics. The average price for a unit of "pharma quality' (top quality Western or Korean produced) HGH is around 3 USD to $8 USD. The HGH can be combined with a lower dosage of testosterone from your physician. It's quite difficult to receive a prescription in many nations. There are a variety of forms of HGH and you must inject them all in a safe manner or should you overdose the vein, or swell the nerve, or accidentally inject it into your eye or nose, it is possible to become blind if not yet from the endless writhing that you've been doing to your sexually sexy.

It's about HGH and a low amount of testosterone to maintain your testosterone levels at natural levels. A few steroid addicts engage in blasting, also known as the process of cruising. It is when they raise their levels of testosterone far over normal levels, causing them to rise and then lower the levels back a little bit, which is known as crusing. It's extremely risky even when they're doing the tests for blood levels, but there are many who live their lives in this way. Others who use steroids go through an "cycle" of period of time, then they completely fall off their unnatural levels with these post-cycle replacement medications to restore natural testosterone levels and reduce the levels of estrogen. It's essential to have an after-cycle program that will help you avoid loss of all gains in muscle to maintain testosterone levels, and to avoid nasty adverse effects, such as Gynecomastia or 7 Litres of MILK Bitchin' tits.

These kinds of programs that are more serious, I'm unable to give advice since I've written this, it's a program produces high natural levels testosterone, and high levels HGH not natural, however are subject to a physician's study.

If you are relying on other people to sell you stuff it goes up in price in relation to the number of grubby manhands and hot Thai or Chinese lucky-fortune-waving-catzpawz that have touched it before it arrived in yours. It is impossible to tell whether it's genuine. It is possible to lose thousands of pounds and kilograms of cheesy poop $$$##$$%%$$$ If you do not find the genuine bargain. Srsly.

I'm not able to discuss this subject since I'm not knowledgeable much to be able to speak about it...but be careful...be mindful of the potential dangers. If there's no way to know the substance you're injecting, or paying to get it, that's not the best location to be in.

Make sure to use only those that you can identify as expolicemen women, or even exsportsstars. It's not hard to get along in the case of child celebrity when you are able and stare at their pathetic infant faces, which are all deformed because of the cromagnolia Agromenly Disease that is caused by huge doses of HGH in the past. Don't want to be in the same conversation as your Ex-child star dealer in the gymnasium.

--Fuk My slow trans sibling's great Ape clit! What's this thing you bought me Heidi? The gear is all bright and dirty. Why is that?

It's a good thing, don't be concerned.

Yes, I'm trusting you but can you look at these slender fists? They could tear the decaying and rotten ass from a massive six-foot Australian fruit bats at night, which quietly moves by means of ecological location.

So can I, Heidi, so can I.

If my cholesterol is even so skewed that it's tilting in the wrong direction on your body, damn it, I'll ensure that you're feeling like you're having your period You're tempted to wash the blood stained laundry, however, it's pouring rain outside, your boyfriend's decomposing corpse is boiling in a pot in your kitchen, your inlaws are coming around and you're consuming meth. descend when it's like the lights go out, and you notice the hairs on the ends of my fingers beginning to echo.

....know what I'm talking about ?!!? Heidi You large German Ape dick...I I will destroy you.

If you're as me, who is standing in the line at the grocery store but all you're thinking about is how you want to relax and get an excellent clean and some beating right now, it's a good idea to poke your ears, and then listen carefully because I have some suggestions specially to help people like you. Make sure to pin up yer huge cat ears and take a deep breath when I spit some words through your the plugholes of your giant cat ears.

We just got back from the gym! Doing bench presses as high as 100, but this was done with the help of my Korean trainer Hyoung. After that, I did a dumbbell chest press until 22.5 kgs. I was doing around 8 sets, up to about 15 reps, but not as much at the higher weight. It's finally time to use the chest press machine. Are you getting it? The workout session .... kinda boring!

That's how life goes as. You GOTTA JUST SUCK IT UP. Do not be like GIANT Cylops, who got pounded on the cheek by a tiny man. Fuuuuk. This guy was just one-fifth his size, and yet a long-time cyclops let himself open. Be sure to guard yourself against your most vulnerable areas. Do not think...just take action. Simply get to work. Create a checklist and make sure you get your meals eaten, the medications taken, and workouts blasted out. Do your best to improve. Do not just focus on your upper body, make sure to work also on your legs.

Take a look at everything I write, and follow my recommendations throughout this series, starting with volume 3 and to. DON'T READ BOOKS 1 AND 2 IF YOU CAN HELP IT COS THEY ARE BORING AS FUK. It is me alone who can show you precisely what program I'm following. Others will offer you an ebook for between 15 and 30 dollars and they don't even include photographs of their progress. What exactly can you possibly be able to follow this?

Now, on to the progress I've made. I don't really see an improvement in my chest and the appearance is thin, despite an increase in muscle beneath. Therefore, I'm reverting back to drinking 5 litres of water a day is a good way to burn fat down. I'm hoping that it keeps some of the fat off, while allowing the possibility of massive growth.

I would suggest that if you plan to take steroids and hormones, consult a reputable physician. Any doctor can do. The UK majority of top consults are doctors origins from India, Pakistan and Africa in general, so if uncertain, go directly to the sources. If you're located in Asia most appropriate place to is South Korea, Seoul. Send me an email if located in this area. I'll tell you the best way to go and the best place to get steroidal medication legally if You are likely to be over 30 yrs old.

The doctor I trust just wrote me telling me they're changing the definition of my low testosterone jab. I'm required to visit for the jab within around a week. The doctor is really great physician. An expert. The testosterone hormone is a human growth hormone CIALIS. This is the type of doctor that you'll need for your particular case. He was hard to come across. In part 2 and 1, I was having difficulties finding a doctor who could prescribe HGH since most doctors do not have any knowledge about the procedure. In the case of extremely special clinics I went to it was very complicated and complex and it took several months to get anything. When they finally could offer the information, they could not give you the dosage you'd get! Daaaammmmnnnn.

It was a very special experience okay. They were waiting in line with Aspbergers as well as my slow sister who gave me a slap in the butt, and one of them put a spoon into my face. The great doctor was hidden from view. Doctor Batman. It was in plain view because...he was my very first and regular doctor. Who could have imagined that?

I was searching Seoul for clinics to combat ageing. Kiss my ass Special Clinics! It was an enormous and sweet waste of my time and I was nearly sucked in the face by Asbergers

My-slow-sister, as well as those specially designed anti-aging services with a total cost of 2.2 million KRW or 2.200 USD for ten weeks of treatment with an unconfirmed dose. Don't get something fancy, simply go to a regular doctor, and they will take care of you and you will be happy through a basic check of your blood, a quick glance over and look inside your pants. Not like these raging anti-aging clinics..................... Faaak dat, big pappa is outta here!! !

It is now time to receive an anti-aging treatment I need to get in form to make angry heads explode in rage at the sight of Shwarzneggar version number T4. However, at the moment only what I have is a massive stomach and a few newbie gains in strength but not enough muscles- that's not enough for all the work I've done!

The past few days have been few blissful days since I first started taking my HGH.

The main thing it's been able to help with is the relaxing sleep provides you with and an excellent quality sleeping. We haven't observed any other side effects as of so far. The expected timeframe is one month, or perhaps several months for the effects to take effect, therefore it's not uncommon.

This is a bit odd because I believe I've spent a lot of time and effort on this course, and have having gotten plenty of support and guidance from two trainers, and with the doc on chemical issues .....and but .....I am still thinking there's a million things to ask and I'm unsure how hard I'm working enough? If I work harder, do I suffer injuries? Actually, I don't have an concept. I have had a bit of shoulder pain that was a phantom, so this might be a sign to not to do too much? If I head to the gym, I'm finished in one hour however, I train seven days a each week. Is that a sign that one hour is sufficient? Confused. As a cat sips the semi-skimmed milk bowl I'm wondering what else there is to life? Are I on the right path, or is there something I am missing? some thing?

It's impossible to buy this type of knowledge into the harder areas of elite athletics. What do you think Mr. Natural Hero Bodybuilder Star will describe his struggles in this or another area or the best way to handle the effects of overtraining? He's not going to say he's consuming all the right things training hard, doing a lot of exercise and doing the same thing or do this. The truth is that I think that if there isn't a knowledgeable trainer or friend before you begin, you'll likely give up before finishing your program. It is likely to happen within the first 6 months. If you come across Andre The Giant, Jaws or Arnold I'm betting if you approach them, they'll honestly say it's best to work with a coach to aid you with bodybuilding, because in the absence of a trainer, you're likely be unable to begin lifting weights and challenging your body. Or you may even overtrain.

One good benefit of working six days a week is that I eat 12 before and after work out meals, which has to be positive because it gives me more opportunities to take up the protein! Most people are of the opinion that after work-out meals are crucial for the development of muscles. Yet, do I need to drink a cup of coffee instead of pushing it at the gym more during each workout? I can't talk to any of my three idols because I'm sure two are gone and Arnold has been busy with filmmaking.

Today, I'm on whole milk. I'm considering drinking 6 litres of semi-skimmed MILK per day in order to lower the calories. Every carton contains 900mls but they're not sold in litres. It is 6 calories per day, which is 382 calories. = 2300 calories. With a massive mass. 1200 calories provides the total 3500 calories a day. Just did some searching on the internet. 20 times weight in pounds provides the number of calories needed for a diet that is bulking. Based on this formula, 20 180lbs (my weight) equals 3600. Also, if I take six litres of milk as well as some significant weight (SM) powder, I'll need an extra bit. You could try 5 litres semi-skimmed, and 3 SM, which equals 2000 x 1800 = 3800. It should give you sufficient calories, and somewhat easier to drink maybe as just five 5 litres. A third scoop of real mass won't taste great, but it's one or a 1 litre of semi skimmed. Both aren't appealing however 5 litres are much more manageable.

This is

1. There is less fat in the milk than the previous time with the full milk as well as

2. A lot less calories too.

To see the progress of this plan during the coming weeks. Even though I'm a fidgeter and might alter the plan before having enough time to fully put it into practice.

I measured myself and measured the weight of 83 kg. There are also several kgs of milk in my stomach. I'm expecting. Also, if we say the 81kgs, I've lost 10kg in the span of the space of six months. It's possible that 3kgs could be muscles. That would be 7 kgs of fat at an approximate estimate. It was sort of preordained since I was consuming much more calories than my body can convert into muscles.

It is now possible to compare this to the next six weeks that will take me through the end of January, 2016. The way I'm going to go is to follow a more fat and calorific eating plan from now on, and I am able to assess how much weight, muscles and fat I gained over the time.

I'd definitely read about it and understood that I ought to aim for 500 calories, or about my average daily intake which is more than the is required for my typical daily intake that was around 2700 calories in my initial weight. But, I was unaware the prospect of having a large excess was likely to result in an issue as the article states/promises in the following paragraphs.

Perhaps, I was thinking that I was unique and would put on the bulk of muscle instead of fat. However, I realize the huge surplus did not work and am going to try this more practical and less frenzied strategy. If I do find some small amounts of 'roids functioning properly, then it is at least clear I'm capable of consuming 5800 calories with no hassle and know how to accomplish it.

This isn't something to be taken lightly. I'm an autistic person and I speak a couple of languages. My sister who is slow to speak doesn't understand even a word and doesn't understand what to do with having 5800 calories. That's what I do. I've tried it before...with the force of MILK...WHOLE MILK.

In the event that I'm hungry, along with my grandmother, I'll never want to miss a meal under the magnificent desert starry skies in the night...roasting her in the smoky charcoal campfire of a turkey. Just hope those ape dick desert nomads don't turn up to my feast as through desert convention it is very impolite to refuse them sanctuary...everything in life is set against me...the desert, the nomads, work colleagues, home environment, the gym opening times, the worldwide health monopoly and all but a few doctors, my bank account and my own frikkin' body...with these forces ranged against me how can I ever hope to become a giant chested ape dick that could smash the shit out of bonobos asshole just by dropping my giant acromegalised massive boned hand on its belly which is as soft as a calves-foreskin causing it to crap itself.

The article mentioned below, they're affirming that you can build 1kg of muscle per month, with just a bit of fat, and over the course of an entire year it's about 12kg of muscle. From this, I could infer a long future target. Perhaps I'll be muscular with a weight of around 95kg by the close of 2016. However, the article does not cover the effect of HGH as well as test...so could be a superior result. Is it possible to achieve 100 kilograms? It seems like a good amount to target towards.

Just did a small amount of study about testosterone. According to online forums, including the unofficial bruvscience knowledge center that if you consume under 500mgs testosterone in a week, you're inefficient. In contrast there were a few people who were taking 250 mgs per week, and one was able to achieve amazing results, so he recorded. I've checked and confirmed that the information I received was

Chapter 2: DEPO-testosterone injection of 250 mg with

-HCG 500 IU.

The HCG is primarily responsible for preventing the size of your nuts from decreasing by keeping testosterone production at a natural. This means that we are able to overlook the HCG and declare that I'm taking an average of 125 mg testosterone per week this isn't much considering an average steroid cycle would be 500mg per week. As for the effects, they tend to show up within a time span of 3-8 weeks.

In addition, there's HGH currently at 3 units per day, but could soon hit 4 units. That is where the bodybuilding benefits begin to manifest. It takes around three weeks before you feel the effects, and it is likely that from the between the middle and the close of December, I am likely to look to see if something can kick-start either a bit or possibly.

If you're anything as me, you've experienced an entire month of intense bodybuilding and sleepy like a baby, and have spent all your money to buy your doctor's wife costly clothing and accessories, you'll be wondering when those serious best pharma drawer medications will finally start making a difference? When???! !

If I'm not paying top dollars for sexual sex with the hope that a big girl isn't going to get pregnant or give me something I'm not looking for and I'm able to enter without condom only to discover that my incredibly mean-spirited my mofo's slow-sister hasn't taught me anything regarding sex and ed. I've used up all my cash on no gain. If she was lying about this then what else was she lying about? It could be that girls have babies in the event that they have sexual relations with dogs? I am thinking to myself with a stunned look on my stunned face.

After you pass out due to the loss of blood, you turn and you see the family physician behind you, sitting on your shoulders with his hands in the air and a "phooaaaaaw! expression on his face. the doctor gets ready to deliver another huge blast with a divining stick that is covered in Leaches with a mutant that wasn't even in the prescription form.

The main thing I want to say is that I'm not looking for excessively positive or a pleasant feeling to begin since I believe I could take these drugs to last for a long time, but when they're too pleasant, it won't be ideal as it will result in a violent crash someday, something I definitely don't want. It would be great to know that HGH can heal my mysterious shoulder pain. It would be wonderful that my sweet sister wouldn't tell me lies. It would be wonderful that I did not be fighting so much to earn an ounce of respect this place. It would be wonderful for things to be slightly easier. Let me share some new information to share with you.

That's bodybuilding. IT's HaRd... RealLY HaRD. SrsLy...frikkin' hrd.

Bodybuilding is said to be an entire lifestyle and I definitely see the benefits. It is something more of a full-time Korean occupation. This is a job that's continuous throughout the day, and you don't get longer than a couple of hours off as it's always important to watch the food you eat. There aren't many holiday days and you must work the grind if you wish to achieve to succeed. This is an extremely competitive workplace.

This is another reason to pick Korea as a place to start your training for bodybuilding if you want to travel elsewhere for the initial few months of your training. Another option is Thailand but it is possible to become distracted by the gorgeous temperatures and skip going to the exercise facility. In Korea many people are working at their best, and you shouldn't think that you're not getting enough exercise if doing your exercise and have the strict schedule of sleeping.

I am prone to moving about a lot, and must learn to find places to exercise, completely and eating a flexible diet. How am I supposed to get the right amount of HGH and testosterone from these locations, if they aren't there is Korea? WTF? This isn't possible. It will be quite a hassle, in the event that it's even feasible considering the huge trouble I experienced when trying to find it. It is true that bodybuilding is an all-time job.

If you're anything like me, and have written hundreds of ebooks on topics that you and no others like immigration law, distance education or learning a language, Hitler timing travel lezzer porn with erotic sex as well as generalized Asian-German blonde Cajun porn is for you. You'll want to read this article carefully or maybe smack yourself with a huge oily syringe filled with HGH. Although I usually hit my HGH into my stomach, however I've observed at the very least a expert say that it's supposed to become intramuscular. It's even completely autistic. Aussie slow sister who is fluent in 9 languages. Languages desertsands delay in defcon 5 intravenously! WTF? In venously...jesus Christ? Who is Jesus Christ? Sure, only Jesus Christ, the SON of God could do this?

Do they want to murder people, make jobs in the industry of medicine or even create giants and krakens in the bodybuilding community as they're supposed to? Fuck me hrdr. The pro athletes are serious mofos...injecting HGH into the veins? What? I don't even know how to identify a vein when my gym bunny opened her mind and said to me that I should help myself, and to 'just get deep!. While I smoked meth for 15 years, I just put the drug up my nose Hitler way. Blasting HGH through the veins? Woah.

I'm planning to consult my physician to see if they could smack some of my voice box and then take me to the karaoke bar and test if that helps me become more of a singer...I believe it will work...but as we all know, I'm not going to be able to do it in real life. Shame. The possibilities are limitless...

Returned from the gym without PT only by myself. Did

2 sets of shrugs,

Three pretty poor biceps exercises, which included around 10 to 15kg and

triceps pull down.

I got a good feeling of energy at the end, and did not feel fatigued because I took a cup of coffee! It's a good thing that caffeine is helpful, but when comparing the things I accomplished today by myself, to the work I get from the help of a coach and specifically the psycho trainer, it's somewhat sloppy.

Psycho trainer has left the premises. I shared my experiences of this trainer who was first-class in my second installment. He helped me to not fear massive weights, and taught me how to have fun exercising. Through the joy of deadlifting and turning weightlifting into a fitness test game.

Just returned of My Korean English conversation exchange. I'm supposed to be studying Korean and I do not yet know whether I'll be staying or not. I'm still waiting to get begun. I'm feeling a little empty. I'd like to stay and not leave, but I must find a job or begin the business. Have been thinking of the possibility of starting a business from home however, it is not going well in the present. I've looked into a few sites, however it appears to be common knowledge that the prices are extremely current and therefore not the best time to invest in. You can also buy a property and lease individual units through airbandb and earn a decent amount, however in the event that you do not manage to let the units out it could cost you many hundreds of thousands of dollars because rent prices are excessive and you need to make a huge deposit. There are a ton of suggestions for barspew ideas, that aren't completely insane, but a lot of them are.

All I can guarantee is that will continue to work in this BODYBUILDING project no matter what. The world may take my toys, however I'm not giving up for this toy vehicle. I'm not sure the reason behind this or whether it's improving my experience of life in any way However, there should be a reason behind why I decided to start it. Maybe it was the right one which is why I'm determined to continue giving it everything I can.

As if the dead, rotten out R2D2 smug roid head that has Princess Leah within his thoughts with his mouth full of with 'roids, joints stuffed full of sand, and ears overflowing with shit, I'm going to continue fighting this battle as that stubborn old goat Count Dogo in Star Wars...no whatever silly, shit and hurtful things people think of his loose hair, wispy facial hair and goth gear...I'll continue to fight to defend the Empire until the dumb dodo's brain can be revived from the ashes.

I keep a mental mnemonic within my brain that is REFeree. It reminds me that I'm always required to make sure I'm taking my Roids or exercising, as well as food. As I'm no longer drinking 6 millilitres of milk anymore, it's easy to keep track of food or drink. But in the past, it was difficult to not pay attention for several hours. Sometimes I'd realize I'd lost my post-workout beverage or had reached the point of exhaustion yet to drink two three litres of milk. It's worked for me.

If you're me and find that the majority of the best concepts you've have ever had were just plain crazy shut your eyes, don your glasses, pour your cat a cup of semi-skimmed milk, remove another cigarette from the pack and remove that layer of smoke: get ready for a soak in the warm of the natural buzz.

I just returned from the training. It was an interesting workout. So had my caffeine and my creatine. In order to get creatine I'm using concret creatine. I'm not sure if it's any good or not, as I'm doing a lot of other medications in the meantime to determine how it works...either is the case, it was fascinating.

When I walked into the gym, and thought immediately what have they accomplished to beat! The music is incredible. It was then that I thought I'll think about it for just a minute...I am in the middle of a high. Was it a mistake to take 1.5 tablets of caffeine, instead of half (cos I fractured them all into half). And then I thought, well I had one half of a cup today and I didn't really seem like a weird experience as the one I had just taken.

Therefore, I don't know what the reason is, but I felt very high.

I tried the squat, and I believe I did around 100 kgs or even 110 pounds. That's quite a bit greater than the normal amount and could mean that I did around 70-80 kgs. It was then that I noticed an enormous pumping through my legs during the squats. I was exhausted, yet still very high. Hyoung I was hearing her say 'Hey! Hey! Hey! Okay, I'm you're not done yet, but OK!' I performed lunges only with the bar. It was a struggle since my legs were dead. There was a T-bar row that is in the smith machine. You raise the bar with your legs. Also, my legs were dead, so there was nothing on the bar. I don't know exactly what was going in the background. The legs don't seem as tired. I'm not sure if it had a high during the time I was doing squats or whether I actually used too much energy in the very first exercise and didn't have enough remaining energy for the next two workouts.

My gym, as well as my personal trainer costs approximately 600,000 KRW or USD/month which is higher than what I'd like to invest. For the longer term, I'm searching for a gym that is free as well as a gym that is less expensive. I placed an advertisement on Craig's List and came across one person who was studying in Seoul National University who says I could use the facilities at the school which is why I'm planning test it. I also found a lot of users, too, however they do not appear to be able to access an exercise facility or have any knowledge of any nearby. There many gyms available within this region. True, however many of them are costly and others are extremely difficult to locate except if you're Korean. Korean.

Today's food intake is pretty good. I've recently had my 3rd litre of whole milk that has a serious weight. I still have entire milk in the refrigerator and I have consumed four litres full of whole milk, two massive mass as well as 2 scoops of protein. It's 3600 calories. This is prior to getting into the semi-skimmed.

Cor Interesting fact. We didn't even know about that. It's a fascinating nugget.

You'll be able to experience the essentials of the Krakken application! You can't resist the temptation to make the real-life monster Karak'ken quite boring, do I? Sure, it's boring. That's life. The only way to succeed is to work just like Spiderman in order to achieve success.

A nice feature of Seoul is that they have plenty of activity on the meetup.com website. There is a wonderful Korean study group located in Gangnam. The best part is that I am able to walk thereas it's situated on one of the roads that is part of Gangnam highway. It isn't clear what the highway is, but it's got Gangnam station on one side and Sinnhyeon, I believe on the other. The group meets at the Dropbox café. The groups are of around four people so you really get to get to know each other. It is a 45 minute chat. minutes on whatever topic and you switch tables after that. If you wish to get to know people, you need to visit them numerous times. They're very friendly and warm individuals. It's great that they can be found each day of the week therefore there is a lot opportunities. The majority of them are in for the age group 20-30. There are some hilariously good characters in there.

Most hilarious was one Korean who was from Georgia, USA who insisted on breaking out into an spontaneous hip-hop. We were discussing the fact that some Americans do not know much regarding geography. When we were talking about France and the fact that they use French in France He was yelling "wow! I had no idea'. It seems like he was playing his own game as he should be aware of French people who speak French but not English however it was hilarious. He concluded by rapping a hilarious rap. It's quite unusual considering that majority of Koreans seem to be completely different and tend to be more serious and committed. However, this was probably the most enjoyable conversation I've had in every time I was to Korea and had numerous amusing conversations with a variety of individuals.

Another reason I was thinking of is that I experienced difficulties when using the injector pen for the HGH. It occurred to me that using the inside of the bic biro I could just use that to press the plunger. I'm thinking I sucked myself a little additional jab in the morning and maybe that's the reason I was high today?

If your situation is similar to mine, and constantly in a condition of sluggishness with regards to the cost of your physical energy at the gym, you could learn from my book and experiment with the HGH and testosterone mix appears to be working quite well. It could be too effective, maybe. I'm excited by its possibility.

It was decided to have some time off today as I'm going to the gym next week on the campus of Seoul National University. I was exhausted and I was unable to sleep until 3 am. It was likely that I was overexcited because of the same chemical problem that I experienced earlier. Following my HGH dose again, I was completely exhausted, and I would say energetic and sluggish. In further research it is apparent that HGH may cause this lethargic sensation as one of the impacts. In my previous post, I prefer it to my usual state of mind. It's like having a enormous amount of fatigue but it's still enjoyable and calm. It's similar to getting anti-anxiety medications at no cost, in addition to the HGH and I'll complain. If you experience any social interaction, for instance the time I chatted with some

Korean acquaintances for a couple of hours today, I was extremely wired. I'm hoping it doesn't impact my sleeping habits in the future. The only reason that I've slept more soundly recently is due to the effects of HGH, which makes it problem with it.

My legs are completely in a state of death this morning. This was definitely a great workout today.

Another effect that comes with HGH could cause you to not feel needing to eat much, which I've had this today. But I believe I've consumed the calories I need for today, so it's all good.

If you're anything like me, searching for great fitness tips, you won't go off from examining a number of the articles on the website in the following. He seems to have a lot of advice and has written a really interesting article on HGH here http://johndoebodybuilding.com/?s=hgh

This is the greatest piece I've read on HGH. It's the only one I've read that highlights some things that I've noticed also concerning HGH. The author advises you to increase dosages gradually. Be careful not to jump into the highest dose, or you could suffer an extremely unpleasant experience, like the one the ones he mentions that can cause you to be sick for days and days. In addition, he mentions my lethargy I've had.

It was only recently that I realized the Friday evening class was when I was able to pull out some hundred dollars to cover the cost of the following lesson, thinking it was a Monday. About 6 hours later that I realized that it wasn't the beginning of a new week. It was Friday. I was paid, was not conscious of what I was doing when I was at work. Therefore, I believe you have to be cautious with this as you could be in autopilot. It doesn't really matter, however there are other situations where it can cause danger, such as when you're in a car or running. It is possible to imagine you going straight through trees or crashing off the edge of a mountain. It's not you, but someone who is high on HGH and wrapped in pleasant thinking as they go through the trees. SO WATCH WHERE YER GOIN ON DIS STUFF!!! This being said, I love this type of sensation and will accept the feeling and enjoy the experience!

I'm not very hungry. For me, this isn't an issue since I'm able to get the milk and the powder down well. If the powder was solids, I would think that this would cause more problems.

I know now what huge fatigue I've experienced since that's what John Doe said he suffered from and is one of the main reasons John Doe doesn't take HGH nowadays. He was however going as high as 8 units the times. That can be a very high dosage. In addition, he did not even slow get to that point, He just went from 4 units to 8 at once, which means you're taking the risk of experiencing sudden adverse negative effects.

He recommends very minimal dosages or cycles of testosterone. He seems to be saying at least 100mg every week that's what I'm discussing, is something is considered to be very efficient. That's also great news!

The doctor warns that faces may become changed by HGH. I looked for this on Google and couldn't locate any other instances of it however it is something you should be conscious of and research when you're concerned about it, which you ought to be. In my case, the slight alterations in my face shouldn't cause any problems, so I don't worry about it. It's supposed to happen only at extremely large doses, like more than eight units per day, and when you use it for a long time. However, there are not any set guidelines for the product and you'll never have a clue. It's possible that something could go wrong, but most likely, it isn't. In any case, the risk associated are low with HGH are substantially lower than typical steroid usage, however it's important to consider the perspective.

It's a bit like those who can't consume a lot of milk and therefore cannot adhere to the GOMAD plan because they suffer from digestive or other issues with having milk. For me, I'm drink only frikkin milk, and I can take it with no problem. If I consumed the exact amount of calories as solid food I can imagine that I'd be suffering from constipation. This is because if you eat plenty of food, and you don't drink plenty of fluids, you could be constipated quite easily. Everyone is unique.

This writer also points out that HGH could allow bodybuilders consume a lot of food and maintain their perfect body and that's why it could be harmful for overall health as people take full benefits of this. In higher dosages, it could cause the stomach to stick out, for whatever reason and it can cause some serious discomfort. The doctor recommends not exceeding four units daily It seems.

I'm off to the gym right now.

Just took two concret creatine pulls, and half of a caffeine tab. My legs seem inactive. I'm physically tired However, now that the coffee kicks in and I'm feeling slightly more energetic. Still, I feel tired and sluggish, however. It's like I'm always struggling to breathe or exhaling very loudly. Because I'm getting fatter, my acid reflex, or the heatburn issue has returned. in the last couple of days, I've had trouble getting sleep. It's now days 10 on the HGH and testing 'cycle' or programme. Therefore, the results shouldn't begin until. It could take up to three weeks to allow the HGH and blood tests to show up it is believed.

So I just go to the gym but it was shut. It was a typical Monday.

The most interesting part was the fact that I felt my shoulders were very relaxed. Normally, I have to be able to rest my shoulders, and especially the left shoulder that gets higher as I work. Today, however, I could completely drop my shoulders as if I were being in an chair, and it was so soothing.

The same thing happened last night as I attended "Open College," an amazing club in Seoul that lets people take part in various cool courses including three-dimensional printing and role plays theology, psychology trip, justice home camps, and a host of incredibly bizarre and amazing as well as projects I'm unable to think of currently. Yesterday, I was to the club for the English chat class, which I offer five days each week. I sitting on one of the large cozy chairs there and then fell asleep.

Today, I was able to experience a few kinds of "tracers". You think that you see someone walking alongside you. But actually it's the tree or another object and you see it as a slow-moving that has tracer traces appearing off of the surface. This was a pleasant HGH rush. The HGH buzz can dull your senses and cause fatigue However, it's quite comfortable. It makes the annoying stuff less irritating and you be more relaxed about your surroundings. You feel somewhat sexually attractive or even a bit enthralled and it can be reflected into others, meaning it's like you're enjoying a good buzz. It's a great aspect. Of course, you'll always have that massive insanity to overcome.

After walking to the gym, my legs and body are more sore...I suppose I'm going to try some stretching out this morning if I have the motivation to try it.

I went to the Co-ex Building in Samseung Station this evening to meet my former dance partner. It was a pleasure to dance with as well as an intriguing lady. It was a pleasure to dance with her but it was a shame that she decided for pilates.

It's precisely 6 weeks I would guess. It's time to review. In essence, I notice an extra bit of muscles on my arms, and that's the only thing I see. Also, I noticed that my abs went away under the additional 10kgs of mostly fat I've added to my weight.

I'm attempting to present an accurate picture of how the program will work out if I do the maximum amount of effort and utilize training, time, nutrition, rest and most importantly HGH and testosterone in an extremely low dosage, as well as caffeine and creatine tablets.

I just measured myself and it reads 85kg! This means I was 83kgs just a few days back. It's not a problem, but I'm now bringing my calories back to 3800. So, it's a good thing. This is a concern since the extra weight will need to be mostly the fat. As far as I know, without steroids it is normal to add 1kg of muscle every month unless your an amateur like me and in that case, you could make more. If you're using steroids, it is possible to gain between 3 and 5kgs of muscle per month (maybe as much as 10kgs in a month on some steroids cycles- the only information I have about it is via browsing forums on the internet etc). The fact is, I just begun using steroids and would have likely not had negative effects for 10 days. However, I was able to add a significant amount in the first few days of their kick, since I am an inexperienced user, I am able to gain more weight, which is known in the scientific community as beginner gains.

According to some reports, it is believed that adding HGH to testosterone is akin to the act of throwing gasoline on the fire...your body explodes! In all likelihood, I'm not overstating things and that's the way I've been told to believe by reading online threads on forums. There are only a handful of sites I've come across that actually tell you precisely what you should do, like John Doe's link above. The users, therefore, are lost.

It's difficult to stay glum and stress excessively when you've got the Anvil of HGH depression settling in your brain...just lucky that I was able to take the tablets of caffeine, and I'd probably have been in bed in the morning, unable to type these things. My traps growing, but not my lats or those muscles that run along the sides of my rib cage. They are the ones that need to grow and I want my entire back to expand. It's a long process, however I want to start seeing some improvement before December's end or in the next 4 weeks.

Now I'm going to put to some tunes and perform some exercises since I'm not able to go to the exercise studio. Well, did thatand it was very helpful. It is recommended to do stretching before and after exercising. I've noticed that it really helps. I'm currently out until 6pm...maybe can take some sleep. Trouble is, I'm now getting the caffeine... I can't fall asleep... and even when I am using the force of HGH.

I received the following email message from my physician. The site JohnDoebodybuilding suggested Cialis as a medication intended meant to be used for ED but in reality, it is an enhancement of mood as well as increasing blood flow and many other beneficial effects. The doctor has provided some details about Cialis, including the various doses. I'm planning to take some next Friday, when I head back to the clinic for another testosterone shot. The Cialis I'm thinking is pretty nice...I enjoy an erection that is spontaneous, like my own, in general enjoyable. But it isn't without risk. impossible if you're doing it close to the person you are dancing with. There have been issues when it came to this throughout my life I'll wait and test that...but in general, it's nice to be able to keep your dick when you're just strolling around in order to lighten the monotony.

There are several interesting threads on the internet. There is a suggestion that not many users make use of HGH because of the cost. Will learn more about it later.

Going to the gym right now. I'm back, and it's surely better for all of us. You'll feel great going to the fitness center. While in the gym, the music has a fantastic sound. I felt great throughout the workout and by the end, I thought I had a lot more left in my tank. I just had a post-workout breakfast of milk, and the weight loss was well-received.

Today's exercise was back. I did

Romanian deadlifts up to 120kgs, but I managed to do the exercise for around 8 repetitions which means I am much stronger than I was previously as I was able to perform one deadlift of the weight, if I recall right, however now I'm doing about 8-

10 reps after doing several sets leading towards it. Doing a pyramid set of this.

After that, I did some barbell rows. think the weight was not enough, around 60kgs when you maxed out.

Then I did the lat machine pull downs for 50kgs. I'm thinking four or five sets of around 12 repetitions.

Feeling exhausted while I worked out However, I've found my groove back and I'm feeling great!

I'm going to look into the forums for steroid users and read more. Given how great it felt today, I think there is no need to take the Cialis stuff...can't envision how wonderful it will make me be if I incorporate it to my mix. It is my goal to be cautious that I do not be too happy. If I feel that way, it could mean that you'll have to go down which is why I like to not be feeling too great so that you do not have to get rid of anything. Therefore, a slightly good feeling is the best

I could ever wish to be. I'm planning to purchase the most affordable generic Cialis pills at 20 grams, and break it up into eighths or quarters. You can then take only as much as I am able for a few minutes to experience a minimal effect.

The other thing I noticed is that now that I've become larger and more slender, I am proving to attract more women and receive more compliments. It could be some steroid have this effect which is probably more likely. However, it's a nice thing.

It's costly. My money goes to training and meds. I was planning washing my pants that I usually wear, but then I realized that I didn't be wearing anything. I'm in need of new clothes, but by the time of my departure, I'll need to invest an additional few hundred dollars or pounds for HGH. I'm not sure what they're pricing in the meantime, but it was the last time they had medical doctors and expenses for blood tests. I went to the movie on a Friday night and paid dinner which was around 70 USD or 70,000 KRW. It was impossible to eat the majority of it, and my stomach became bloated throughout the screening. The good thing about Korean cinemas is that the tables are placed in between seats to ensure that you're not completely stuffed up. In any case, the budget will be tight, and I'll definitely need to fit into the Cialis purchase in because it's been highly recommended.

Chapter 3: only find this out WFT?

In my school days, I was always apathetic about sports and would need to have a quick line for a boost prior to matches. Smoking made me miserablely inactive. Now, that I can get a perfectly healthy moderate high that includes traces and pumps, as well as spontaneous boners as well as heightened enjoyment of music, increased concentration, feelings of happiness, a better appearance as well as more attractive, and a greater health, and generally sexually attractive.

The only thing I heard was to not make use of steroids. It's actually not quite as straightforward as it seems, is the case? I believe these are suitable drugs and they will also assist you in finding to fight aging, etc.

Now that I think about it, I recall many times ago, reading the huge Sunday Times newspaper over a lengthy breakfast on a Sunday and learning about the American children who were growing into huge head roids. They were presented in the article as if they did it to get bigger and be constantly covered in acne, and engaging in fights. The journalist was missing the whole point and completely did not inform me in a timely manner and in a way that was unfortunate. The reason people were taking the steroids was that they had fun and it made exercising a lot of fun. It seems to me that the growing massive is due to the byproduct. If you can do it naturally, it is possible to avoid the negative side effects and a range of steroids while still getting massive (through HGH, but maybe)...anyway it's what I'm trying to discover through my researchezzz!

The truth is, I'd had been taking this drug several years ago, if I'd realized beforehand. Better late than never, but shit what a giant ape dick fucking-my-slow-sister oversight.

The HGH can make you the ultimate sex-attracting magnet. NO joke. You attract people with a pleasant manner. It may become annoying at a certain time, like when you begin with auto-boners. In the meantime, you've spotted an vintage WWII German lady who walks by and gives an attractive minx look and then she claims she gave you an enormous amount of money. ......

I just got back from training. It was a good day, I think...hard to believe! I only managed to lift 40kgs using the shoulder press in the smith machine or less than this. This doesn't appear as though it's high enough. However, the amazing part is that even with the drugs within my system, it sounded great and wasn't dull in any way. It's now clear what's the secrets of gym-goers and the athletes. What makes it so interesting at the gym, while whenever I would go, it was utterly boring. Since they're all taking one kind of drug or hormone, like TRT, HGH perhaps greater than others. .... It's simple and really nice... It's very satisfying to be working out on substances. This is an amazing feeling.

Doing shoulder presses with dumbells weighing around 12 kg.

And finally, the overhead press machine that weighs approximately 30kgs.

Finally, it gets trapped in the smith machine, and then the triceps will pull downwards. I felt a nice lift in the upper physique.

Are doing deeper research into HGH. Many people suggest that you divide the dosage if you're taking more than four units. Other people suggest it's not a big deal. Additionally, I found out in another publication that six units are what is needed to build muscle, and it's what I'm trying to achieve. I'm not able to commit to divide units (ie daily two injections) thus I'll just aim to get up to four units a day, and then slowly increase it to several units per week, until I reach six units. In essence, there's no definitive solutions and a lot of contradicting data available. What I know is that bodybuilders with professional training (who are also afflicted with a sour roid stomachs) can take as much as 60 to 70 units per week, and do it 3 times a each week for a total in the range of 20 units. Amounts of more than four units at one time is considered to be an inefficient use of energy, as many claim the liver is unable to process more than 4 units at one period of. So, it is recommended to split doses: one at the beginning of the day and another after lunch. But according to this reasoning, the professionals who take doses of 20 units one time, or even a whole day are wasting cash. There is many contradicting data. Perhaps it is best to break the dos in the event of taking four units if you're able to bear the burden. You can also try the trial and error method yourself to determine if this makes any difference to your personal situation.

I'm not able to imagine what negative side effects could be in a dose that is really high (although I'm guessing that 70 units doesn't sound like a lotas it's only 10 units per day) However, visually you will see the digestive problems experienced by the top bodybuilders who some attribute to HGH while others attribute this to excessive consumption of carbohydrates or a fumbling using insulin. There is no answer. However, one suggestion I think is an ideal idea is working up to 4 units per day and observe how that develops over time before adding more. The advantages to the mind at 4 units are worth the effort. It's hard to say what the physical benefits as of yet.

The costs are slowly increasing and I'm having to cover rent for this week. Christmas is coming up and I don't have enough money to spend on a night out. Need to purchase my new medicine on Friday. So it's becoming very frustrating and difficult.

My English coworkers from the project said they were amazed at my muscle mass and that at the very least certain gains can be seen. The muscles are definitely bigger however they aren't remarkable yet, and obviously I am a big tummy. The doctors said that I looked more youthful, stronger, and slimmer than I was previously. OR similar to that. They were basically saying that they you looked healthier in comparison to prior to. In my opinion, it's strange because I was thinner in the past. However, I believe what the real meaning was I appeared better and definitely the HGH can make you appear better looking in some manner since it alters the appearance of your skin. John Doe bodybuilding's article on HGH was a reference to this and said that the face looks more attractive when you use HGH.

I'm beginning to notice my back starting to form. As I was stretching on the machine, I could feel my sides. I could also sense the lats beginning get a shape, which is essential for a V-shaped back.

Talked to Hyoung in the gym while the trainer was working with another. He's planning on ordering an additional mass. This one seems to have vanished so quickly. I'm sure it's nearing the finish line, yet I bought the pack recently.

I have eaten three liters of milk as well as 3 scoops of seriously massive mass this morning which leaves two milk litres to go. It's all semi-skimmed milk.

There's no time of calm when you're a part of this frikkin programme. I've been fumbling around in search of money to cover the cost of my doctor's visit this Friday. Was trying to figure out the amount he's going to cost me. Thus, I received 3 vials the last time I took HGH Each one contains 7.5 mg. Each is 22.5 units. If I decide to consume six units per day, I've calculated that this amount approximately

1400 USD per month, which I can't pay for. If I reduce it down to five units, I'll possibly manage it at around 1100 USD for a month. Theoretically, I could manage this, so I'm going try to do that.

The main mass appears located at the bottom of the package. Shit. This didn't last very much time! What is it that I should accomplish with my diet today. My main issue is that I require the carbs in the Serious Mass. One serving of Serious Mass consisting of two spoons with the trowel that is included in the bag are around 1200 calories as well as 250 grams of carbohydrates. The calories can obtain from milk, but the carbs will be more difficult. You could have a slice of bread, however that could seem a little difficult because I'm not carrying butter or other food items to put on the bread. Do not tell me to purchase an ice cube that can be spread at the shop...can't even think about doing this.

I'm looking for at least three thousand calories. I need at least 400g of carbs as well as 200g of protein at least. This means I'll suffer from a lack of mass at least for the next week. If I purchase WHOLE milk which contains higher calories than skimmed milk, in 6 litres I could receive: 6 x600equals 3600 calories. Then 50x6 = 300. Six 30 x 180g = 180g protein. 6 x 50 equals 300g of carbs. However, I'll get a lot of fat that I had been not avoiding previously, however in order to get the more calories, I'm likely to require whole milk.

If I only drink six total litres of whole milk per day, I'll get nearly all I require, so I will continue with this strange regimen again even though I've never found any Serious Mass fat burner. There's a different, less expensive powder in my cupboard, so I can add a small amount of it into my diet to boost the proteins if I'm able to find the time. There is an limit on the amount of fucking around that it is possible to engage in. It's never over.

Shit. I was hitting myself using the Bi-Biro to release the plunger, and wanted to determine 5 units. There is not a measurement in the vial. It's also difficult to read on the back that of the pen...problem is, it's quite a distance from my stomach to my eyes, and the vial is somewhat small. I'm guessing I could be able to give myself 8 units or more. Today I'm feeling quite tired. It's good that I've eaten breakfast and consumed my coffee and creatine as well as headed to the gym in the near future to get my day going well.

Let me tell you an intriguing aspect of this HGH. JohnDoebodybuilding said HGH can make your skin look more attractive over your face (and that it may cause you to be deformed later, however that's a different story I didn't find any information about). Also, when I visited the gym last week, one of the women from the gym walked up to the counter at the front and, looking at my face she said, 'you're gorgeous'. It was quite unusual, considering that it's a formal high-end health facility for families and not a massage establishment. HGH has this fascinating result on skin.

Absolutely misdosed this morning However, it feels very nice very nice. It's probably a good thing. The cost is approximately 30 USD per day. At the moment, I think that it's worth it...but I'm always on the lookout to see sides and come downs...so do not let it seem too good.

I'm barely weeping as my ears keep popping...mmmhhh I need to go for an fitness. It is now clear why exercising can be so enjoyable. It was a great day today. Felt nice again. Doing chest press and chest press using dumbells, and then using the machine for chest pressing. I felt exhausted at the end of my workout, so I tried another set of at least the most reps I could do.

Wow! I just had an uneasy feeling in my stomach completely in the middle of nowhere. This was not a great experience. It seems like I've felt too relaxed lately. I'm going to have to be on guard for the situation. Do not want any crash thoughts to be on my horizon.

After a long night out, which was fine. One aspect of my life I will definitely finish is this ridiculous program. I'm completely unconcerned about the rest of my life. This is likely to be a lonely, boring experience since I will need to forgo everything else to go for it. I won't have the money for a lot of different events. I will not be able to pay for the other classes. I'll most likely eat out. I'm going to take all the way and give all that I've to offer. Do everything else.

I'm back from training. The last couple of days have been very rough. It's been quite depressing compared to last week or as. Perhaps the jab test did not work? I'll get another one on Monday. This seems to be the most plausible reason. I thought about the ridiculous amount of work it takes for bodybuilding. There is never a chance to unwind. The powder is gone Then you suddenly have to complete a whole different diet regimen to take in. If you are doing something different during the day, it becomes apparent that you've never consumed anything. It's a horrible feeling and you're still required to go to the gym each day. You begin to become extremely fat. Like you're about 25-30% body fat now I'm guessing, which means it's time to reconsider changing your entire diet program. You set it up only to find that you've ran out of protein and you're unable to accomplish it. After that, the frikkin' pills make up the bulk of your income, and there's no money to spend it on a trip. This never ends. And then you stare at yourself and wonder. What's the point of all that? It's still pretty like before, and in fact slightly worse because in the beginning I was abs-focused and am now obese. How long will it take me be able to benefit from this? And what is the best time to find a groove in this area where I'm not constantly worrying about it every single day and having to rework the entire routine every single day or at least every couple of days. It's never ending.

There are only two positives to this: fitness is actually enjoyable when you're on the drugs. This is all there is!

Today, as usual, I completed my usual Thursday routine. The workout was okay. And then I concluded with a deadlift, observing the heights I could go to and adding more weights each time. Finally I got up 135kgs. This is 295lbs. I am about 187 pounds. A great deadlift, or a regular deadlift should have a weight of around 1.5 times your body weight and that's about 280 pounds, it means I'm barely more than a normal deadlift for someone of my weight. At least this is improvement. Also, it's a lot of amusement adding weights to your lifting and getting yourself motivated to lift the weight.

The rest of my day was just a shaky and a shabby day. It's snowing, and I don't have enough cash to purchase the perfect warm jacket since I'm spending my entire budget on other necessities. It has been a pleasure to meet nice individuals in Seoul. It's much easier to make friends here than other places, but I do have something to admit. In the end, not too terrible.

We just came back from the surgery of a doctor. The doctor gave me Cialis generic. It is a mood-uplifting hard on the manufacturer with a smile, stating that it's recently been granted patent protection. This was $30 for 8 tabs with 20 mg. I requested that he keep the cost at a minimum of 600 dollars. The doctor then gave me three vials consisting of 22.5mg for each HGH. I also took another dose of testosterone.

This is the problem if you are you take 6 units per day, this is 180 units in a month. One dose of 22.5mg is just 180 dollars! For a month, the price would be 1400 dollars. This is quite a bit and way more than what I could pay for! !

The landlord wants me to stay in 4 units, and that's what I'm likely to be able to pay for. The monthly price for 4 units is 1/3 less, which is less than 1000 USD per month. This is still expensive, however it's manageable in the event that you don't live an existence for some while...shiiiiiit. It's just 4 units which means it's going be less powerful.

If I was given the option to do bodybuilding as normal by taking a large dose of testosterone, I'd take the shot, as this HGH does not appear to be robust enough at present, but as I'm taking the route prescribed by my doctor, it's not an choice. So, I'm coming back on the 18th to get my second testosterone dose. I've got 3 and a half vials remaining and I think that's about

70 units for 14 days. This is five units per day. I'm guessing I've got enough to get 5 units daily, I'll take it! !

Cor Just returned from the fitness center. My azz hurts bad! But it's not that bad. However, my back is completely exhausted. As I walked back I was unable to figure out the reason for what was happening. I was unable to walk. I've never had this issue prior to this. I was performing squats but my problem was that it totally destroyed my mid and lower part parts of my back. It was necessary to lie down several times. I was walking for five minutes home, and I was receiving some odd glances. I was just about to fall asleep immediately. After returning home, I've sat in bed for about an hour in total slumber. My back is still tired however, my legs seem normal. They're just exhausted. It's a little odd that.

Today, I did squats with 100 pounds around and was incredibly difficult. I didn't remember to take the tablets for coffee. I had a double espresso however it did not have any effect. As my thighs and upper back are above horizontal during the squat when I am at my lowest spot, at the same time as that huge load, I'm not able to lift it to the top again, or do not have enough strength to get it back to the top. It seems like my leg strength isn't quite there as of yet.

In any case, afterward I performed lunges using about 30kgs, and then a T-bars rolled in the smith machine once more at a low mass. Weird. I'm currently in my seventh week, and I'm performing a pathetic amount of leg exercises. I don't understand why this is like my legs aren't growing quickly. Do I need to do two legs a day?

It's like my speed has slowed down this morning.

Doctors say I'm basically in the 4 unit range for the duration of time. Besides, I'm unable to pay anything more than 5. And even for that, it's a sign that I'm unable to consume. Perhaps at this dosage, it's enough to make muscle, which is exactly what JohnDoebodybuilding suggests. But, another source recommends minimum 6 units to build body. You can't go wrong, just wait and pray. There's nothing I could make. In addition, I have to figure out an avenue to earn an increase in income. I had planned on operating a guesthouse but it I think this isn't an ideal time to start this type of venture. I might try to get an ongoing job, but the paperwork has been making me feel uneasy. I need to decide shortly. Financially, the first part of this month is going to be very difficult.

I sucked my 20mg Cialis generic pill into eight pieces...well it's very chunky and unevenly sized and I was able to cut it in seven pieces...but I did find it to taste good and wasn't as sweet as the drug dealers speed...yuuuuuaakk.

It's only a couple of mgs to test to see if it has any effects. If not, you can take many more in the near future.

Did some searching on an steroids site. It was extremely interesting. They said HGH can be injected either into either the muscles or in the fat to alter the bio-availability and half-life. It isn't clear which is the better option, however on their figures it looks like they're about similar. There is a wealth of useful information on their website about HGH, however they offer an advertisement for an untrue product. authentic, and is not pharma-grade HGH, so beware of this! They can really fool users into false feelings of security by providing high quality info, but they then direct you to a poor product. This is hilarious and clever since they warn you against counterfeit HGH and then the supplement they refer to isn't real HGH however it's supplemented HGH that is administered through a spray. It is not going to generate large quantities of

HGH when compared to the 'pharma grade' or actual HGH which must be administered. This is why this subject is so complex and difficult to obtain information about HGH and to know the price is the right price to pay, etc.

However, I'm not at all, and I imagine this plan stretching until the end of January or Feb. before I will see tangible results from the HGH. Woooowww...cool but I've just realized that I had a swelling in my right hand earlier this morning. This can be good since that's the HGH aspect, but it was very tolerable and even quite relaxing and shows that it is at least a sign that the HGH has been doing some thing. It was almost as if I felt my hands megoargogelomanic as they were changing into heavy hands of stone.

If I'm experiencing those sides, then I am benefitting. If I examine my hands, I can see that they appear to be larger and swollen. However, I've been drinking my caffeine and coffee before, so the positive sensation is being a result of the caffeine high.

Two liters of whole milk this morning as approximately 24 litres were delivered today, and I've started my diet of all milk. I am feeling very overweight.

I'm back from a workout and taking another two litres of whole milk today. It was just a matter of doing my workout by myself this morning.

Three set of arm exercises that I'd consider to be pretty weak. I was able to do 8 kgs in dumbbell raises. I also did a preacher curls of 15kgs for the Then just an unweighted bar sitting up.

And then shrugs off with dumbells of 15kg and 40kg triceps pull-downs. The pump did work but that's a good thing. However, it's extremely frustrating that whenever I'm doing the workouts by myself, I can't even get myself into performing the weights that are heavy. I just don't want to or do not have the time to do doing it. If I'm working out with my trainer, it's always one hour. There is no cardio. Does this sound like a great plan? It's hard to say. It's simply to keep going. In the end, I'll be able to learn in one manner or another.

It is quite unpleasant to be drinking milk at this point. If you are just looking to consume a litre of milk, with a little powder, it is straightforward. If you need to consume 2 liters of milk it's not a good idea since one liter of liquid is already enough to fill your stomach and it's not something you want to drink any further.

It's another point that's low. A bodybuilder who stares at the mirror and sees 30 % body fat, with no muscle type of low. What are the freaking monster outcomes you promised me, oh my slow azzburger anally redone? Have you been causing me to cry again your sly witch?

Go to Bangbae around 3 pm to participate in the English chat, and we'll check out how it goes... typically, it brings me joy. There are a number of administrative tasks to sort out this weekend mostly involving money. Need to determine the best way to go about it or the things I'll be able to cut. Shitty shit, shit. It's a lot of fucking sh*t. Fkkaarrrrhzzz!! !

Then I came up with a vague strategy. It's like being trapped in a dark hole by this at the moment. Costs of this mean that there's no space to do something else. However, I'd like to give HGH an opportunity to prove the potential of it. My sister in law has assured me that if I adhere to the plan, I'll never experience regrets and that by the middle of the month of January, I'll begin to see huge gains. Therefore, I'm putting all my faith on her.

I'm going to give up everything else until January 15th, my date for renewal of my visa. This is approximately 10 weeks from now, which will be the 5th of December. It will provide me with the time to commit and then I'll be able to make certain drastic changes in case it does not work or if I'm unable to go without a break. It is my goal to be massive, and even if I'm making significant progress, I'll continue to suffer because it is the most secure and most effective way to increase my size is to use HGH instead of other kinds of cycles, which can be more prone to danger with greater fluctuations. You can't even get steroids even if you'd like to, unless you reside in a specific area.

The other option to reduce costs would be to go to a different gym, as well as cut down on individual training, but at the moment I'm not sure if that would work as an answer considering the fact that I'm physically lazy even with these dosages of medicine, I'd never be able to improvements. Therefore, I'm stuck in this regimen as well as this gym at the moment.

However, this doesn't sound good. I've been considering alternatives. I.e. go somewhere else or try something different. I'm sick of all this rubbish. Are you interested? You're right, I've written the stuff I've written, and given it all for more than two months. I've made some progress (at at least, the HGH is good, and I've been able to get the occasional quality nap as well as some gains in strength) However, will I be able to handle another two months like this? I'm in need of some relief however I am unable to take on anything else during the remaining two months. What can I do?

I went to the gym that is located in my apartment and $40 per each month. The gym is small and appears to are equipped to perform similar tasks, but their dumbells are probably only upwards of 10 or 15 kgs while another gym can go as high as 30 kgs. Correction: they can reach 30kgsHowever, the deadlift bar does not come with a lot of plates. There was thirty pounds already in it, as well as nothing else about that I could find. There's a couple of small plates for the bench press. So perhaps it's going to be a possibility. If I weren't tired of individual training lately, I would not even think about it as a possibility, however since I'm bored of the gym I am in, I'm thinking that I might give it a go. It is possible that I will be able to meet new friends in the gym, and since I'm located right next to the gym location, it might be much more enjoyable. There are two PT classes left that I've booked, and I may be required to relocate at the beginning of the next week.

Even though the PT exercises appear to be more effective that what I am able to do alone, due to economic reasons I'm not given many options. If I train alone, I am able to take longer than an hour and you should be able to more up for the loss. If I am doing PT exercises, it's typically the first workout which really hurts me then it becomes simple, so if I simply take a whole caffeinated tab instead of all of it, I'll be able to make up the different. You can also conduct more studies and discover ways I can improve my exercise.

But the main risk is that, if I begin working out completely by myself, I am most likely to be performing such pathetically slow exercises that fade after a few days of utter no-things. Perhaps, I overtrain and become injured.

WTF. I'm looking for a different environment and also the cash. I'll give it a test on Tuesday, when I work my shoulders independently.

Today, there are two parts in this program that don't look well. The only thing that is solid is the roids portion. I received my HGH injection this morning. Then I got several times during the early morning to feel quite pleasantly and with a fascinatingly bloated hand. Particularly the right hand. It wasn't uncomfortable whatsoever. The sensation was truly enjoyable.

The fitness aspect isn't optimal due to the danger switching gyms, and being forced only work out by myself within a small, unequipped fitness center. There was no staff on hand, so I'm not certain which way to be handled.

Food isn't very good. I'm downing my fourth cup of milk this morning, which isn't pleasant to drink. I will have to wait until the middle of next week before my PT gives me the most powerful mass powder he's ordered. Once I've left the gym, I amn't going be able to purchase the powder again. It's a bit up and uncomfortable. This will end up being one gallon of milk every day, and that's it in the near future as long as I'm not able to find another provider.

There is a reason why you cut down on the steroid doses so that you'll have the money for all the PT as well as food that you'll need. This is certainly true, however the researchers conducted a research study using testosterone. They discovered that individuals who exercised and did not take steroids gained muscles, while those that did not exercise or took roids only gained a great deal. This is the reason I'm in favor of the drugs. If I weren't taking the steroids it would be boring to attend the gym that I would not have been there to begin with. They are therefore essential! This is to say, they are essential because I love them. I find it fascinating to experiment with this HGH substance that provides an altered state of consciousness that it is said to cause amazing effects...so I'm not letting go from this baby. It's essential, as I require them to help get my body moving. HGH is among the most intriguing things that happen that happens to us. It's amazing to me that I was unaware of the hormone until just a few months back.

Every smart drug is excellent. Like Modafinil. However, the problem with all that legal speed is that you are still experiencing weird and bizarre mental symptoms including paranoia, as the effect is just too powerful. The need to go off the drug at some point. In the case of HGH you will only experience an altered state of consciousness, and some other magical physical manifestations (hopefully). However, who knows what additional impact it may have when you know more about it. I'd like to be there for some time in order to start playing around with it better and understand more about the technology. There could be innovative ways of using the technology that haven't been discovered.

So, I had a few PT lessons scheduled this week. I'm likely to pull them out and begin on my own personal exercise plan on the next day. Because I will use less weight and smaller volume, I am planning to increase my frequency and do greater sets and reps.

In the in the morning and at night, doing twice every day, in order in order to increase the frequency to make up the huge loss in quantity (although when possible, will strive to achieve 75% of my one's personal records, although I would guess that 30-40% may be possible in terms of plates that I could add).

All this is just nonsense talking. The fitness center is crowded but there's no space for the deadlift...so I'll try it at the beginning of the day tomorrow to test it out.

I've just done some research to determine whether high frequency, low-weight training for bodybuilding could build muscle as much as weights with heavy loads and it appears it does. A technique called HST. From my perspective, it's because it requires longer at the gym for the same results. If you lift many times, this could lead to injuries, I'd think. However, as I'm not able to choose, I'm just going to try this in an enormous way. Therefore, I will definitely start to see what happens I am so excited! There is no choice for me on the matter as I'm saving 600 dollars each month. I hope that I can learn through this journey.

I've just completed a lot of digging around and have completely revamped the program for workouts. It's quite intense and does not have enough sleep within it. However, browsing the web I found that there are people who exercise twice per day, six days per week. Some are even training seven each week! A man even has the owner of his gym open to the day on Christmas! He works out every day. He's a beast.

However, the weights are likely be far lower than I'm expecting and I'm planning to do the sets and reps more slowly. But they will not take long, but they'll simply blasted out in a kind of random fashion, at a moderate speed because that's how I train. That's it! ....we are going to wait and see! Then I will be completely dependent on myself...no further individual training. However, I have coffee as well as the fitness center is located opposite, and it shouldn't be a problem to find it.

We just got back from the neighborhood fitness center. They do have the equipment they need, but the place is crowded with Korean OAPs who aren't to be very happy. However, it was a good experience and just 20 meters away from my door.

That's precisely what I practiced during the morning exercise and plan to do similarly during the later afternoon. My back was stiff from doing squats earlier in the week. First, I tried:

deadlift 10 x 40kgs deadlift 10 kgs x 40 kgs, 10 kgs x 70 kgs

Barbell row two sets of 10 with a lower weight because my back was fatigued. I couldn't hold the simple posture without weight.

Pull down the lats at 50 kgs. 3 sets. 15 repetitions.

There are a few shrugs, triceps and some gidd.

Was planning to do squats and actually my back was just exhausted from the week before and I was not able to perform more. This isn't surprising, but the back seems completely dead after Leg exercises on Friday. I'll be back to the gym in the afternoon about 2 pm when I hope the OAPs will take time to rest at home, and perform the same exercise again. Just finished my second boring tasteful litre of full milk. It tastes bland and heavy to me. However, it's calories, so I'm simply drinking it.

Recently, I contacted a person via the Korean messaging app called "kakaotalk" and requested she call the gym to inform them that I had put 40 dollars at the desk to pay for membership fees (Korean 40000

Won is the same as 40 USD, therefore it is easiest to simply use the word dollars even though I'm non American). The gym was empty as I walked in, and a lot of people do not speak English particularly OAPs. I it was just me leaving my cash on the counter. Korea is very isolated, and oddly, you may encounter strange reactions when you enter Korea for a foreigner however, young people tend to be very welcoming, perhaps more than any other place on the planet. There not as many teenagers living in Korea since it's extremely expensive and demanding procedure to have kids, so it is less of a concern for people. The government actually has an official wedding schedule that follows the strict guidelines. Therefore, for the first year after your marriage, you're expected to live in your home, before you start having kids. If you don't follow that then it's not normal, I suppose.

This is a stressful time and many people avoid this altogether. However, I don't blame the people who don't want children, because although they will be loved by you, but it's not a guarantee that everything goes well. Personally, I'd be satisfied with just a couple of pets of my own! This is pure love. Funny thing is, I'm not sure if I'm yet ready for this step because I don't even know where I'm in my life, and therefore I can't buy an animal as I believe it is necessary to live in a permanent location before doing this. It's not fair to take on the responsibility of any animal without being completely prepared to take on the responsibility. If the homestay allows pets I'd definitely take it on as it will be a great pleasure having a pet around. Actually, I have just sent an email to me my Homestay agent to find out the homestays where there are dogs allowed. I might look into this.

I've observed that many Koreans do not particularly enjoy pets, but it's permissible to have a small pet. If you own a bigger pet, people can be scared by dogs. Let's be able to see.

Okay, just returned from the gym after my second workout today. The second session was similar to the first one. My back was very fatigued. It was...

Chapter 4: A couple of sets of deadlift at about 70

Barbell row was almost impossible since by this point my back was too fatigued, however I managed to do some sets at around 15kg

I was able to perform the lat pulldown in the exact same way that I had done before with about 60 pounds. This is proof that when I exercise by myself I'm not capable of letting myself fail. It's just not my thing to get myself into the habit. My body doesn't want me to expend that much energy. Therefore, doing two times a day could be the only option to get me to utilize all of my potential. This means that I can still snooze while working outs, however since I'm working out twice I am more likely to achieve outcomes.

And then some lunges, 10kgs, 3 groups of 20. The exercise was not very effective, however my back was strong enough to let me do nothing more. Because of the same reason, I could not do squats, I just didn't have the strength.

A few weak shrugs from the smith machine, approximately 40 kgs. It's due to the fact that I had been able to get upwards to 100 kgs using the straps and trainer. However, I was doing dumbbell shrugs in the morning and I'm hoping that is a good sign.

Triceps - repeat the same exercise that you did in the previous morning.

The issue I am able to notice is that while my back feels dead, however my entire body does not feel as if that was my intention to defeat. However, it's an excellent beginning so I'll maintain it. If I get energy and pumped up in the near future, I might attempt crossfit but if I'm still a tiny lazy person who cannot endure running for longer than 50m as it causes me headaches and causes my lungs hurt, I will stay AWAY...but should I be able to get enough medications into my system that keep me motivated, I'll attempt to go out to show the unfit fitness lovers the proper way to get it accomplished...

At the beginning of my own scheduled, low volume intense training that begins at the start of week 8, I am carrying plenty of fat as well as some muscle. It is my expectation that, if everything goes well, I will shed a significant amount of fat, and add additional muscles.

However, at this time I needed to go back to Korea and wasn't able to obtain HGH recommended in any other country. Training with no HGH was not a lot of enjoyable. The workout was fine however it was not fun. Thanks to the HGH it was it was the ideal thing to do at the period of time. It was fun and easy to exercise iron. However, now that I'm returning to my normal boring self. I just lack the drive. Therefore, my project has come into a premature end.

Chapter 5: What is Testosterone?

Testosterone, a potent hormone that is found in females and males in addition to other mammals. It is able to manage sexual desire, improve power and enhance testosterone and sperm production. It can also increase the risk of aggression and competition and also human behaviour.

Red blood cells

Bone density

Functions of sexual and reproductive

Muscle mass

Particularly in males, the testicles are the main source of testosterone. In women, however, there's a lower levels of testosterone. The production of testosterone increases in the early stages of puberty. It then begins slowing down after thirty.

Testosterone is a key component in the formation of semen. This like a milky liquid that aids in the motility of sperm. is among the many reasons which contribute to the demand for sex driving. The hormone is often connected with sex drives and has a significant role to play in the production of sperm. It also affects the size of human bones and muscle in addition to the fact that the fat we find inside our bodies. It produces the red blood cells..

The mood of a male may change due to the testosterone levels.

How is testosterone created

It's a rough flow charts of how visually-oriented learners it is.

As we age, testosterone levels decrease in men. production. This causes the testosterone levels to fall. Stress or chronic illness could reduce testosterone production. certain examples are listed below.

Alcoholism

Kidney disease

AIDS

The liver has cirrhosis.

A low Libido

Testosterone is in the adrenal glands located on the upper part of our kidneys.but 95percent of them is produced in the testicles of our body.

The three kinds of testosterone.

Free testosterone

SHBG Bound testosterone

Testosterone bound by albumin

Testosterone is primarily produced by the testicles. Testes are the place where Ledge cells convert cholesterol to testosterone.

The majority of testosterone production occurs in the testicles. The testosterone that is created forms a bond with sexhormone binding globulin SHBG and it is no longer useful.

Free testosterone. The rest of testosterone, is known as FT. About 2 to 3 percent of the total testosterone in good condition for bioavailability and usage.

The most significant hormone that circulates in the in the brain .we are able to receive signals regarding the amount of testosterone that is present and the rate at which it's produced.

Testosterone Need for our Body

What are the things our bodies to use testosterone?

Testosterone hormone is an androgen. It creates male characteristics within the body. Testosterone is made in the following location.

Andrenal glands

(Located just above the kidneys, both women and men)

Testes in men

Ovaries in women

The testosterone levels in men are higher than testosterone within their bodies as compared to women. If either testosterone levels drop there could be negative signs.

Testosterone in Men & Women

Which is the most effective way to use testosterone both genders?

Testosterone is the main ingredient responsible for numerous male body during the existence. Testosterone aids in the external and internal organs that aid in male fetus's production. It includes male reproductive organs, including the testicles, and penis.during puberty, testosterone can be the main reason for this.

A deeper voice

Growth spurts

The growth of hair is seen within the pubic area

Underarms and face.

Testosterone also has a role in the functioning of aggression as well as sexual desire. Men require testosterone in order to produce sperm in order to reproduce.

The hormone also performs functions that are common for males and females. The hormone can that stimulates our body to make new sperm to reproduce.

Testosterone role

Testosterone is the most prominent sexual hormone that males use and has a variety of key role, like.

Strength and size of muscles

Sex drive

The penis' development and the testes

The voice becomes more deep as puberty progresses

Production of Sperm

Bone strength and growth

The appearance of the facial and pubic hair begins at puberty.

Testosterone can also aid in helping keep you in a good mood. There could be another reason for the hormone that has not yet been identified.

If you believed that testosterone is only important for men it is wrong. Testosterone is produced by the adrenal gland and the ovaries. The only testosterone-producing male hormone. The hormones can have a significant effect on.

Sexual behavior, including normal libido

Even though the evidence isn't definitive

Bone Strength

Ovarian function

Symptoms of Excess Testosterone

What are the reasons and manifestations of testosterone excess?

A high level of testosterone could create health problems.

Males with high levels of excess T

Particularly, boys who enter puberty known as precocious puberty, might become precocious.

Muscle well developed

Facial hair

Voice deepening

Sexual organs growth

Precocious puberty is often due to a medical condition that is known as a tumor or the congenital adrenal hyperplasia.

The most likely causes for excess testosterone among men are:

Utilizing anabolic steroids

Congenital adrenal hyperplasia

The testicles are a source of tumors, or adrenal glands

High and Low of Testosterone

The testosterone levels are high and low. dose quantity

Nasal sprays, buccal tablets gels, natesto, Axiron creams, underarm solutions which includes patches are all simple to apply, but they must be used often.

Inadvertently, you place children and women at danger of high levels of testosterone.

Because of the extreme and minimal testosterone dosage it causes several adverse side effects associated with TRT.

High levels of exposure to testosterone could result in a depletion of testosterone, and then a transformation into estradiol which is the estrogen hormone. In excess, estrogen may result in breast enlargement and tenderness.

The other side effects of TRT can include:

Acne

Sleep Apnea

Increased RBC

Breasts that are larger

A low sperm count

Testicle shrinkage

What happens to testosterone levels as we age?

Testosterone levels in men usually increase between 20-30. The T levels gradually decrease over the course of his lifetime. The levels of testosterone drop by 1 % every year from age 30 to 40. The lower levels of testosterone tend to be more prevalent among men of older age. We will discuss how the effects of age on men, for example the loss of muscle mass.

Treatment of testosterone imbalances

The treatment of a problem that's creating high or low testosterone levels may help to restore the levels. However, it's not always easy to determine the reason for abnormal testosterone levels.

There are many ways to treat hypogonadism, or low testosterone. Such as

Testosterone injectable

Chapter 6: Testosterone implantable

Patches

Topical gels

Men and women alike can benefit from testosterone treatment. Females can use testosterone therapy for sex drives and decrease impermanence. But, they must possess enough estrogen before starting treatment. It is due to testosterone, which can influence a woman's levels of estrogen.

Replacement therapy for testosterone can trigger negative side effects. This includes

Small testicles

Infertility

Acne

Tenderness of the breasts or an increase in size

A swelling in the extremities of the bottom.

An increase in the amount of red blood cells.

A good time to check in is once a month. it is recommended to check in with your physician while you are undergoing TRT.This helps to make sure that the levels of your medication increase to where they ought to be.

Many older individuals with normal testosterone levels supplement their diet to boost their strength and endurance. The current research, however, does not confirm that testosterone supplements can cause these benefits for men who have healthy testosterone levels.

You can increase your testosterone levels with organic methods.

Increase your testosterone levels by using a natural food choices and nutritious food items like vitamin and herbal supplements can help increase our levels of testosterone. It is recommended to consult with your doctor, whenever possible, if you are experiencing low levels of testosterone. Alternative natural treatments haven't been proven to be more efficient or efficient than conventional testosterone treatment. All the supplements you are taking can interplay with other medications, causing a small side effects.

Testosterone supplements can boost the sex drive of your partner?

When it comes to how lifestyle, depression, medications, and stress may alter your sexual drive The physiology of your body is another element. Testosterone is the most commonly used hormone which increases sexual desire bones, bone density, testosterone production, and muscular mass.

It is possible that you experience less attraction to sexual activity at low levels, or have a hard time performing sexually. Insufficient sexual desire may cause depression, and can affect existing relationships. Are you looking to take action about this?

Insomnia may cause depression and can affect relationships with loved ones.

You want to take action about this .you need to speak with a doctor who is reputable and provide testosterone therapy can help you improve you get sex as many men would do.

As we age, the side effects can be a result of our genes. there are many factors that may cause decreased testosterone, for example.

HIV or AIDS

Tumors from cancer

The testicles are injured

Tumors of the testicle

Disorders of the pituitary

Inflammatory disorders

(such such as sarcoldosis, tuberculosis and sarc)

In the event that your body does not produce sufficient testosterone, it indicates that the condition has resulted in hypogonadism.TRT treatment is typically utilized to treat hypogonadism. But these therapies can also help clarify what the effects of these supplements are.

The low sex drive causes

If testosterone is low, it's the most frequent cause for low levels of sexual drive among males, there could be other reasons.

The low libido is caused by psychological factors issues, such as

Stress

Depression

Problems in a relationship

As well as lower testosterone, sexual desire can decrease due to a variety of physical factors. One of the reasons is:

Being overweight

Utilizing medications (beta blockers, antidepressants, and Oplates)

A chronic illness

Your doctor (health health care) doctor can assist you to identify the root of the lack of sexual attraction. If they believe that psychological issues could be contributing to the problem, they may suggest therapy.

Natural cures for T levels rising

The treatment for Testosterone isn't suitable appropriate for all. It is also possible to use natural solutions. are readily available to consider trying.

Increase your exercise This will naturally and automatically raises your T-level.

Have a longer sleep time of 6 - 7 hours in one night.

The stress you experience in your daily life can be reduced and learn about methods to manage stress.

Include potassium-rich foods in your diet, such as beets and bananas as well as spinach.

Potassium assists in T level synthesizing.

Zinc is found as a treatment in aiding in regulating the serum T levels for males.

Reduce the amount of sugar you consume during your daily routine.

It is recommended to add zinc into your daily diet through whole grain foods and shellfish. You can also supplement your diet if it is possible.

Will Milk Decrease Testosterone Levels?

It can also help maintain men's healthy bones. Children and women are both recommending drink milk to improve their well-being. Choose milk that is enhanced by vitamin D. Vitamin D in milk can help maintain testosterone levels at a balanced level. Therefore, choose a low-fat and skim milk.

What is the testosterone requirement to be in your body?

Although testosterone is a the hormone of men and women which is associated with libido in men it is present at birth in both sexes. In females, it is a factor in sexual desire as well as physical strength, and boosts the energy level also. In males, this is a way of storing the beginning stages of sexual growth and help to maintain the health of a man throughout their the course of his life.

Particularly, the testosterone level of men is highest in his early years. The hormone is believed to be a key factor in many areas, such as

Life style of sexuality

Physical health

Storage of fat

Production of red blood cells

Bone

Muscle mass

Most people notice that once they reach 30 years of age gradually testosterone levels begin to decrease naturally. In contrast, a stop in testosterone production or a drastic decrease could cause symptoms of low testosterone.

The drastic reduction in testosterone levels can result in:

Body hair loss

Increased body fat

Inability to achieve an erection

The strength of the muscles has diminished

Fatigue

Depression, stress or even depression

Disruptions in sleep

The drastic decrease in T levels could be caused by a number different causes. These could be caused by medical conditions, medications adverse effects and other drinking and drugs. The treatment of the root cause may help to reduce your symptoms from T levels.

You should seek advice from an experienced doctor if you encounter low T levels.

Normal testosterone levels

Testosterone levels are normal based upon thyroid functioning, state of protein level, and numerous other variables. It is also known as normal levels of T. It can cause a wide range of men's activities, including

Sex drive

Energetic

Healthful lifestyle

Active mood

A stress-free life

The level of normal, or healthy of testosterone based on T's level must be in the normal range. Based on the latest guidelines from the American Urological Association .a men's testosterone levels that is at or above 300ng/dl an indication of normal man. If the testosterone level is lower then that level, you should diagnose as an insufficient level of testosterone

Around the age around 18 or 19, the testosterone levels reach their highest point before diminishing in later years.

The testosterone levels are low.

When T levels are low, it can indicates that there is a low level of testosterone. This can trigger a number of men's symptoms like

Moodiness

Less energy

Reduced drive to sex

Gain in weight

Depression-like feelings

Immune system is weak

The production of testosterone naturally declines with age but other triggers can cause testosterone levels to decrease.

Chapter 7: The symptoms of low testosterone

Some people are born with conditions that cause lower testosterone levels. If you've suffered with illness or other symptoms, it could cause damage to your testicles, or Ovaries .which produce testosterone.

Men over the age of 50 decrease testosterone production, which leads hormone levels to fall. In addition, stress or a chronic illnesses can affect the production of testosterone. The level of testosterone can decrease as man ages or age. This is why you should follow the US food & Drug FDA advise against testosterone replacement therapy in order to alleviate signs of low testosterone levels due to the age of 50 or lonely.

A low level of testosterone can harm sexual performance. They include.

Infertility

Erectile dysfunction

Impotence

Reduce sexual desire

The low level of Libido

A low testosterone level, in addition to other indications

Motivation is lacking

The change in patterns of sleep

Trouble focusing

Muscle bulk is reduced and increases strength.

Fatigue

Depression

Males with large breasts

Anywhere you suspect that you have felt low testosterone levels, talk to your doctor nearest you to get a an test.

The testosterone levels are low.

Strength is diminished

Gain weight

Atrophication of the muscles

Depression

Changes in emotions

Drive low sex

Erectile dysfunction

12 indicators of low testosterone

Low-sex drive

Blood counts are low.

Semen levels at the low

Increased body fat

Bone mass decrease

The mood changes

Smaller testicle size

Memory is affected

Hair loss

Fatigue

Problems with getting an erection

Muscle mass loss

Low-sex drive

The libido of men is the most important factor in sexual drive. Testosterone has a crucial to play in sex drives in males. If you have a low level of T, is likely to experience greater decline in desire to get sexual relations.

Blood counts are low.

All over the body, red blood cells are a source of oxygen and nutrition. The blood count test is a test that checks the level of your blood as per the guidelines set by CBC

Low semen volume

The testosterone plays an important part in the creation of sperm, most likely to be a milky liquid which helps in the motility of the sperm. In ejaculation, people with a the lowest T levels decrease the amount of semen they produce.

Body fat gain

Men with low T levels can also cause an rise in body fat. Sometimes, it can cause gynecomastia to increase or the breast tissue gets larger. This is believed to be caused by the imbalance of testosterone and estrogen among men.

Dietary supplements can reduce testosterone

Testosterone is one the principal sex hormones that are found for humans as well as other mammals. Men produce higher levels of testosterone in addition to being an essential hormone for males testosterone helps growth in muscle mass, the body's hair and bone mass and helps to increase reproductive capacity.

Certain foods could interfere with this process, disrupting the hormonal balance individuals concerned regarding their testosterone levels might decide to stay clear of the following meals and diets.

Soya products

Mint

Certain fats

Pastries, breads, desserts and cakes

Dairy products

Alcohol

Licorice root

Insufficiency of testosterone

Obesity

Arthritis or asthma

Treatment for cancer

Foods that can help increase the Low T Level

People who are suffering from low testosterone might have the ability to increase the amount of testosterone by eating food and sustaining a regular diet or specific foods like fish and ginger, seafood as well as some fruits and vegetables.

Testosterone is the most well-known male sex hormone, which plays an essential role in the sexual process, fertility and bone health, as well as muscle mass

Between 1 and 2 percent each year, a person's testosterone levels decrease naturally as they the advancing years. The lifestyle and health conditions can alter elements that influence the amount of testosterone within the body.

In particular, in young age, the effects of medical treatment can boost testosterone levels. However, according to our schedule and healthy eating habits, we will also stimulate the body to make more testosterone through a few changes in your lifestyle.

A natural way to increase testosterone

There are many methods to increase testosterone without chemicals, for instance

Doing regular exercise

Avoiding overeating

Sleeping well each evening

A more balanced and healthy eating plan that focuses on fresh food

Top 9 food items that boost testosterone

Oysters

Nuts

Red meat

Beans

Shellfish

Poultry

Plant milk that has been fortified

Cereals

Orange juice

Milk

Dairy products

Fish that is fatty

Fish oil

Trout

Sardines

Herring

Atlantic mackerel

salmon

Ginger

Pomegranates

Extra Virgin Olive Oil

Onions

Leafy green vegetables

Nuts and seeds

Lentils and beans

Whole grain

Foods to stay clear of

Anyone who wants to increase their testosterone levels or volume might want to stay clear of certain foods that can lower testosterone levels.

Frozen

Foods that come in prepackaged containers

Snacks

Foods processed for processing

Canned

Food packaged in plastic

Alcohol

A lot of prepackaged meals, frozen meals and snacks contain processed and refined foods. They are of low nutrition value, and can being high in calories as well as salt, fat as well as sugar.

Most processed foods have a high amounts of Trans fats. These may lower testosterone levels and affect the function of the testicle, as per the results of a 2017 study.

Packaging in plastic or canned drinks and food items which can alter hormone levels.

Boost testosterone

Increased testosterone levels are dependent upon eating a balanced diet and a variety of adjustments to lifestyles and medications are able to boost the immune system.

Also, a person may increase the levels of testosterone in him.

Reduce stress

Making sure you get enough rest

Exercise regularly

Weight losing

Building muscle under training

Ask a doctor for advice on the treatment of testosterone

Summary

Testosterone levels naturally decline with the passage of time, however levels can be affected by health conditions or medication. Speak to a trusted doctor about signs of decreased testosterone.

Certain vegetables, like leafy greens oysters, fish that is fatty, and olive oil can help the body increase the production of testosterone. Vitamin D-rich foods, Zinc, and magnesium are essential to increasing our testosterone levels.

Exercise and stress reduction may also improve the testosterone levels of those with low.

Chapter 8: What is the testosterone powder?

The hormone Testosterone is extremely valuable

Red blood cell production

Sex drive

Bone Strength

Muscle development

It's the most prominent testosterone hormone that men use to sex. Women too produce it however in smaller amounts.

In the beginning of adulthood, in the early years of adulthood, the T level is the most prominent level in your body. At a young age you are, naturally, your T levels to decrease. The levels of testosterone in the body typically peak around the early years of adulthood. As you get older, your testosterone levels decline. The signs could include: levels of testosterone

The emotional changes

Insomnia

Sexual dysfunction

Muscle mass reduced

Today, a lot of products are available that promise to boost the sex drive, energy and strength by increasing testosterone levels.

Before you focus about any of these natural testosterone boosters out what the these powders contain and whether they can benefit your health.

What effects does sexual activity have on the levels of testosterone?

While a low level of testosterone can result in problems with sexual desire and physical performance, having sexual activity can boost the production of testosterone. If you have a lot of sex, can reduce the testosterone levels that you are boosting up.

Summary

Diet and exercise play an vital role in maintaining well-being and healthy hormones. Certain diets and foods include soya, dairy, fats and so on can lower testosterone levels in the body. If you are worried regarding their testosterone levels might be advised to stay clear of these food items.

The hormone testosterone and loss of hair

The relation between testosterone and hair loss is complicated. It is widely believed that men who are bald have higher testosterone levels. However, do they really believe this?

Male pattern baldness or androgenetic Alopecia, affects 50 million males and 30 million females.

Different types of testosterone

Hormone behind hair lossV(DHT)

Hair loss and virility (myths)

DHT or any other condition

Forms of the baldness

Your genes

Testosterone exists in many kinds throughout the body. "Free" is testosterone that isn't bound to any protein found in the body. It's the most commonly used type of testosterone that can be found in the human body.

Hair loss treatments

Transplantation of hair follicles surgically

Minoxidil

Ketoconazole

Treatment with lasers

Women can also experience hair loss caused by androgenic Alopecia. Though testosterone levels tend to be less in females than males but only the loss caused by androgenic hair is enough.

There are many falsehoods regarding bald men. One is the belief that people who suffer from MPB have a higher risk of being viral, and are more testosterone-rich.

Supplements with testosterone can decrease the fertility of men. What are the effects of steroids?

Some men make use of products to look younger and more fit could make it more likely for them to have infertility.

Utilizing certain male-specific products to look more young and healthy, however the use of supplements could increase the risk of having a child.

Young models with muscular bodies show their body in ads that feature models who are new tan or stress of looking like a certain manner that is different in fitness is a great thing.

In the newest superhero film that was recently discovered featuring actors, ads for lingerie that feature young muscular models, the pressure to appear like a certain style or reach an ideal standard of fitness could seem overpowering.

What males may not realize is that a lot of hormone and chemical supplements may be a risk factor for infertility.

Many men are unaware about the risk posed by steroid as a result of the fact that many of these chemicals and hormonal products can raise the risk of fertility issues.

The connection between testosterone and fertility

Dr. declared that there's an enormous importance in male well-being today in combating fatigue, and a rise in energy levels and sexual inclination. The problem is that hormonal medications specifically testosterone, and the derivatives thereof can be used to manage these signs.

While some of the effects of these testosterone-altering drugs may be reversed, experts better advise avoiding anything that can worsen testosterone levels in the body because it can develop stamina.

The experts advise against any activity that can alter your testosterone levels which can increase stamina.

In general, the brain detects testosterone levels in blood, the level it sends to the tests to produce themselves.

It is a typical consequence of the use of testosterone and is one reason that many bodybuilders trim their heads.

The relationship between T and headaches

Make the assumption that there is a relationship

Anyone who's experienced the pain of a cluster or migraine has experienced the intensity of weakness and pain. Did you think about the reason for severe pain or other signs? It could be that hormones are the cause.

People who suffer with migraine and cluster headaches is aware of the severity and discomfort. Are you thinking about why you experience the sudden pain or other signs? The hormone alone could be the cause.

For men, the connection between this hormone and migraine is not clear. There is evidence that suggests low levels of testosterone (low testosterone) could trigger migraines among males. It is necessary to conduct more research to determine whether testosterone therapy could help alleviate headaches.

The connection between testosterone and migraine isn't always as apparent. However, some studies suggest the low testosterone levels could cause migraine attacks in males.

Highlights

Testosterone powder is made up of herbs and various other ingredients.

Testosterone powder comes in a variety of forms and is sold as testosterone boosters that are natural and can improve endurance.

This is a concern concerning a specific ingredients in mix that are commonly used to create testosterone power.

The supplement contains zinc, magnesium, and another healthy ingredient that helps to build bone strength.

Testosterone powder

The majority of the time testosterone is a chemical which is used to:

The production of red blood cells

Sex drive

Bone power

Muscle development

It is the most prominent male sex hormone. Women also make them, but in but in small amounts.

The levels of testosterone within your body typically peak during the early years of your adulthood. As you grow older your testosterone levels will decrease.

Signs of low levels of testosterone could be:

Changes in emotions

Muscle mass is reduced

Sexual dysfunction

Insomnia

A variety of products available claim to boost Vigor drive, sexual sex and muscle-building capacity through the increase of testosterone levels.

Before you purchase an herbal testosterone booster be sure to know the details about testosterone powders as well as their effects on the health of your body.

Prior to purchasing a supplement from a retailer, you should be aware of the ingredients that comprise testosterone powder, as well as whether or not they're beneficial to your health.

The 10 most effective supplements to increase the level of testosterone

Tribulus terrestris

D-Aspartic Acid

Vitamin D

Fenugreek

DHEA

Fenugreek

Zinc

Ginger

Ashwagandha

Shilajit

Tribulus terrestris

Tribulus tribulus is a herb which has been utilized to treat ailments for centuries in the traditional medical field Researchers are studying the levels of testosterone and their effects regarding sexual wellbeing.

D-Aspartic Acid

D-aspartic acid is an organic amino acid that may increase testosterone levels that are too low.

Vitamin D

Vitamin D is an fat-soluble vitamin the body creates after exposure to sunshine. Vitamin D levels could be less for those who live in areas with limited sunshine

Fenugreek

Fenugreek is another herb that can be used.

DHEA (Dehydroepiandrosterone)

Dehydroepiandrosterone (DHEA) is a hormone produced primarily by your adrenal glands.

Zinc

Zinc is a mineral essential which plays a role in over 100 chemical reactions within the body.

Ashwagandha

It is also popularly known as Withania somnifera, Ashwagandha is a plant that is utilized to treat Ayurvedic medical practices.

Ashwagandha is most commonly utilized as an adipogen meaning it assists your body deal with anxiety and stress.

Shilajit

Shilajit is widely used for its use in Ayurvedic treatment. It's a more efficient and safe supplement which can make a significant effect on overall health.

10 Testosterone boosting foods

Foods for high testosterone

Testosterone, which male hormone influences more than just sexual drive. This hormone also is responsible for

Production of Sperm

Bone

Chapter 9: The health of muscles

Hair growth

With age, you may decrease testosterone and also suffer from the effects that are chronic. The condition is known as hypogonadism or testosterone deficiency. So, it is recommended to consult an experienced medical professional. The majority of cases are medically treated in order to stop health issues from occurring.

In general, hormone balance is essential in regulating testosterone levels. That means consuming well-balanced, nutritious and healthy food plan.

Eggs yolks

Tuna

Milk low in fat and vitamin D

Oysters

Beans

Beefs

Fortified cereals

Shellfish

chocolates

zinc

Egg yolks

Another source of vitamin D is of vitamin D.

Even though cholesterol has a bad image, eggs have more vitamins than egg albumin

Tuna

Tuna is high of Vitamin D, which is associated with a longer life span and testosterone production. Tuna is a healthy food with a high protein content as well as low in calories.

Milk low in fat and vitamin D

Milk is an amazing source for protein and calcium.

Women and children are encouraged to drink more milk for better strength and bone health however, milk also helps maintain the strength of men's bones. Vitamin D levels can help keep testosterone levels in check.

Oysters

Zinc is a crucial vitamin during puberty. its actions can be a test for male hormones after the age of adulthood.

The testosterone levels of men who are low benefit from boosting the amount of zinc in their bodies.

Beans

These meals are packed with protein and fiber from plants that keep your heart healthy and may also be beneficial.

In terms of male hormone health, beans can offer more advantages than you thought

Beef

There are health issues concerning the excessive consumption of red meats in the United States.

Certain beef cuts have additional nutrients that may increase the level of testosterone.

Fortified cereals

Eggs aren't the only breakfast item that could assist in decreasing testosterone levels. This is especially beneficial for those who want to measure your cholesterol levels in the blood.

Shellfish

As per the WHO The WHO estimates that it contains an average of 43% daily zinc requirement only in a 3 ounce portion.

If you're diagnosed as having one of the following levels of Testosterone then you'll need testosterone hormone replacement for example:

Injections

Skin patches

Tablets

Pills

Topical gel

Consider making some diet changes to improve overall health. This is and not only treating the low levels of Testosterone.

Consuming foods that are rich in the essential nutrients zinc can aid. Oysters are a good source of zinc. Chicken and red meat also contain zinc. Many food sources of zinc comprise:

Crab

Nuts

Lobster

Beans

Nuts

Whole grain

Men of all ages should try at consuming 11 mg of zinc each day.

Symptoms of low Testosterone

Infertility

Sleep disturbances

Brain fog

Rapid hair loss

Muscle mass is reduced

Body fat is increased

Depression

Breasts that are larger

Tiredness that persists

A decrease in the amount of libido

Sexual activity that has ended

Erectile dysfunction

The changes in your Erections

A lot of these signs could be caused by illnesses or life-style factors. If you experience symptoms take a look at your doctor. They will help determine the root cause of your problem and suggest an appropriate treatment program.

What is the reason for low testosterone levels in young people?

The prevalence of low testosterone is lower for men younger than 30. including.

Utilizing illegal substances

High blood pressure

Anabolic steroids are used to increase muscle mass.

The levels of cholesterol are high.

Overweight

Obese

Alcohol consumption in excess

Obstructive steroids and Oblates

Low testosterone-related conditions could be related to various medical conditions like:

The treatment for cancer is radiation therapy and chemotherapy.

AIDS

Liver illness

Diabetes

Hypothalamic

Pituitary

Tumors

Tissues, cancers or any other condition that affects the testicles. This includes mumps-related inflammation during children

Genetic disorders, like Kallmann syndrome Prader-Willi Syndrome, Klinefelter syndrome and Down syndrome.

Impacts of the T-level on the human body

Testosterone is a key male hormone that is responsible for forming and maintaining masculine characteristics. Females also contain testosterone, however, in small quantities.

The majority of men possess enough testosterone. However, it is also possible for your body to make a small quantity of testosterone. It can cause the condition known as hypogonadism. It can be treated by hormone therapy. This will require a doctor's recommendation . People with normal levels of testosterone are not advised to consider testosterone therapy.

The levels of testosterone affect the men's reproductive system as well as everything else from sexuality to bone and muscle density.

Low Testosterone

Are low-T levels harmful to your overall health?

Low testosterone, sometimes referred to in the form of "low testosterone", is an issue that men suffer from depending on their years of age. Testosterone levels decrease naturally as we the advancing years. Based on the Urological Care Foundation, in the early 1960s, around 20% of males had lower T. As the decade progresses the percentage jumped up to 30 percent for men. When men reach the age of 80 the testosterone levels have dropped by nearly 50 percent.

What causes T levels to drop?

The decline in testosterone levels is normal part of process of aging. The more a man ages and the more depleted his testosterone levels could be. Along with age, a low T level can be caused by a variety of causes.

Tumors, injuries or any other condition that affects the testicles. This includes mumps-related inflammation during children

Genetic diseases such as Kallmann syndrome Prader-Willi Syndrome, Klinefelter syndrome or Down syndrome.

What are the reasons men require T?

Testosterone is a hormone for sex that is made by the testicles of a male. While a child's male body expands, testosterone helps in the development of reproductive organs. In puberty testosterone plays an important function in the physical growth of males who are boys. The hormone grows hair over the facial area, increases muscles, and strengthens the voice. In later years it also is a key factor in the sexual functions of a man.

Strength

Physical energy

Stamina

A decrease in mental aggression

What are the steps to be taken when a test is done?

Prior to the test, your physician might ask you to stop the use of any medication that may influence the levels of testosterone in your body. There are some medications that may increase your testosterone levels include:

Anticonvulsants

Barbiturates

Steroids

Estrogen and or testosterone therapies

If you're currently taking one of the medications listed above ask your physician. They'll ensure that the test results for testosterone are correct.

It is based on your medical condition Your doctor could also take a physical exam. If you're a man and your physician notes that you are male, they can perform the physical exam.

An abnormal weight gain

The breast tissue grows in size

The loss of facial hair

Loss of height

The gynecomastia sign

If you're female If your physician notes the possibility of physical performance, you may

Abnormal hair growth on your lips chin

Atypical facial acne

Thinning hair that's abnormal

Balding in the front

Testosterone test kits at home typically are available through several firms. They make use of saliva or blood sample to measure the level of hormones in your body.

What can I do to treat my T-levels that are abnormal?

Consult your physician regarding testosterone tests if think you might have an abnormality in hormone levels or observe growth issues within your kids.

Many different treatments is available.

The most commonly used treatment for low testosterone levels is the testosterone replacement therapy. TRT can be administered as injections, patches on the skin or a topical gel which is a testosterone-based hormone to replace the testosterone loss out of your body.

The majority of patients find this procedure widespread; TRT is some risky and unwanted side effects like.

Acne

Sleep Apnea

Formation of blood clots

Prostate expansion

Increased likelihood of heart attacks and Stokes

If you're taking supplement, for instance steroids, which normally affect the level of your T, your physician may advise you to discontinue taking the supplements, or offer a substitute

A doctor could also recommend lifestyle modifications that will help you the balance of your T levels like building muscles, working out and weight loss based on the changes in your diet.

Unusual symptoms, like losing weight, loss of hair or acne, if are younger than 40 You may need to examine your testosterone levels in conjunction with reputable health professionals. Tests can aid in the treatment of the underlying medical condition, medical issue or lifestyle in affecting the T production.

Many times, your T levels could be different based upon your age, your drug program, diet or the level of your activity. The test for T may suggest the levels you have are due to the aging process itself or it could be due to additional factors you could personal control and maintain.

Vitamins - Supplements- Herbs

The universe of supplements, vitamins, and herbal remedies

Though some alternatives may be appropriate for men who have low testosterone levels, not all have been thoroughly tested on human beings. Ask your doctor about it if are looking for a particular product or herb. They can provide the most appropriate dose.

In contrast herbal supplements and herbs aid in the production of testosterone by your body. Certain supplements and herbs are designed to alleviate symptoms caused by the absence of T.

Chapter 10: The adverse effects of supplements

The manufacturers of nutritional supplements don't require the approval of The Food and Drug Administration (FDA). The FDA doesn't control the safety or quality of supplements, herbs or supplements. It's possible that a product could be harmful, unreliable or ineffective.

Always seek the advice of a competent physician before attempting a new therapy. Certain treatments can cause severe adverse side effects, or be incompatible by taking medication.

1. Puncturevine (tribulus terrestris)

2. Malaysian ginseng (eurocoma longifolia)

3. Ashwagandha (withanis somnifera)

4. DHEA (Dehydroepiandrosterone)

5. Yohimble (pausinystalia yohimbe)

6. Saw palmetto (serenoa repens)

7. basella alba

8. chrysin (passiflora incarnate)

9. Vitamn D

10. Garlic (allium sativum)

11. Zinc supplementation

12. Pine bark extract (Pinus pinaster)

13. Arginie (L-arginine)

14. Biotin

Consult your doctor

A variety of treatments can be lower testosterone but aren't without risk. Ask your physician regarding treatment options for lower T. They will help to determine what treatments are most suitable for your situation.

Can it be used to treat in conjunction with biotin?

Biotin is an oleosoluble vitamin that belongs to the B vitamin family. It's sometimes referred to in the form of Vitamin H.

Biotin is a mineral that your body requires to convert certain nutrition into energy. Biotin also plays a vital part in maintaining the well-being of your skin, hair and nails.

Can Testosterone Cause Acne?

The Testosterone aids in controlling sexual drive the bone density, fertility and sex drive for males and females.

Thus, testosterone is crucial for health and well-being. Any fluctuations in the hormone could lead to breakouts of acne.

What causes acne caused by testosterone?

Acne is typically thought of as a condition that is exclusively affecting teens. But, many adults struggle with acne all through their lives.

A fluctuation in hormone levels for example testosterone levels could cause acne.

The research has shown that acne sufferers may generate more testosterone than individuals who do not have acne.

How acne develops

Your skin produces the sebum, an oily substance.

A large number of sebaceous glands are located on the hair follicle. The hair follicles can be damaged blocked or clogged with sebum dead skin cells, as well as various other substances.

Testosterone stimulates fat production. The excessive production of testosterone may raise fat production. This can cause an increase in the likelihood of the development of sebaceous glands. The result could cause breakouts of acne.

A lot of people suffer from with a daily breakout of acne as they enter puberty. This is because T levels begins to rise. But hormonal acne may persist into adulthood.

A list of different kinds of acne like

Blackheads

Whiteheads

Pustules

Cysts, nodules and cysts

papules

Blackheads

Blackheads are blocked, open pores. They can be dark-colored.

Whiteheads

Whiteheads have closed, blocked pores. They may also appear as whitish or skin-colored.

Pustules

Pustules are tiny bumps that have been filled by pus.

Cysts, nodules and cysts

Nodules and cysts are large lumps that are under the skin and are very soft.

Papules

These bumps can be painful. They can be red or pink.

Can testosterone trigger acne in women?

Though women aren't producing the same amount of testosterone as males, testosterone could be a factor in acne-related attacks.

The researchers found that 72 percent of acne-prone women were experiencing an increase in orrogen hormones. These include testosterone.

What causes T levels to change?

Testosterone levels change naturally through the course of your life. The level of this hormone increases when you reach puberty. This is true for females and males. The production of testosterone starts to decline at the age of 30.

The levels of female T may rise in ovulation.

The fluctuations in the T levels in women's cycles are tiny compared to fluctuations throughout the course of.

Then, the tumors in the testicle may cause a rise in T levels among men.

Can you find ways to boost to improve the levels of T?

A healthy and balanced lifestyle will help to keep your testosterone levels at a healthy level. Certain habits can help you maintain a healthy testosterone range include:

Exercise regularly

Avoiding corticosteroids

Anabolic steroids

Reduce stress and manage it by adopting healthy habits.

Sleeping enough for at least 7 hours per each night

Eliminate filtered carbohydrates like white rice, white bread, and baked products

Acne cause

Variations in T do not represent the sole reason for acne.

The following elements could contribute to the to the following

1. Cosmetics

2. Genetics

3. Medications

4. The presence of excess bacteria

5. Die diet is rich in refined carbohydrates

Cosmetics

Certain kinds of makeup could block or cause irritation to the pores of your face.

Genetics

If both or one of your parents suffered from pimples and pimples, then you're likely to get the same pimples.

Medications

Certain medicines like corticosteroids and iodides as well as oral steroids may trigger acne.

In excess of bacteria

A specific type of bacteria living on the skin, called Propionibacterium acnes can play a part in the occurrence of acne.

A diet that is high in refined carbohydrates

A diet that is dominated by refined carbs that are rich in sugars, like white bread, sugary cereals and even sweets could cause acne.

What is the best way to treat hormone acne?

The treatments that focus on the hormones of your body are better than other treatments for reducing hormone acne.

The treatment options available here include:

Oral contraceptives

Treatments for the skin

Anti androgen drugs

Contraceptives for oral use (for women)

The ingredient ethinylestradiol can help lessen the acne that is caused by fluctuating hormones during the menstrual cycle.

Treatments for the skin

The topical treatment options are similar to salicylic acid, retinoid or benzoyl peroxide. If gentle, they may help to improve the appearance of acne. However, it may not be effective for treating severe acne.

Anti androgen drugs

Anti-androgen medications such as Spironolactone (Aldactone) helps to regulate testosterone levels, and decrease sebum production.

Strategies to reduce breakouts of acne

The hormonal acne can be hard to control without balance the levels of hormones. If you follow these lifestyle changes can reduce the acne that is caused by it.

Reduce acne, among other things.

Utilize warm water. Avoid rubbing your skin with too much force.

Take off any makeup or other cosmetics completely prior to you go to bed.

When shaving your face, be sure to shave to prevent hair from growing underneath the skin

Cleanse your face two times a every day using a soft, mild cleanser.

Do not touch your face, or scratching your pimples. Your pores will be exposed to more bacterial growth, which could cause acne to get worse.

If you do wear makeup, choose water-based non-pathogenic cosmetics. They will not clog the pores of your skin.

Smoke, stop as smoking increases the chance of developing acne.

If you think that a hormone imbalance is the root cause of acne, then the best approach is to talk about the issue with your physician. They'll be able to identify the reason for your breakout and assist you in determining to determine the most effective solution.

Diet and supplements that work best for hormone-related acne (acne vulgaris)

If you suffer from an acne problem, you're not by yourself. Acne vulgaris, commonly referred to as acne vulgaris can affect 80% of individuals aged between 11 to 30.

While the illness is typically controlled with medication however, other factors such as lifestyle and diet and nutrition can play an important influence in managing and reducing the symptoms.

Acne vulgaris.

Acne vulgaris or acne, can be described as a rashes-like skin condition that causes whiteheads, blackheads and swelling. It can also cause rashes, inflammation of the skin and occasionally deep wounds.

Acne that is severe

Mild acne

Acne moderate

Acne that is severe

Nodules or large inflammatory lesions or both, constant and burning, acne that have not improved following six months of treatment or any other acne that causes severe mental anxiety.

Mild acne

The lesions are non-inflammatory and mild in the case of acne. Or, some inflamed lesions, or both

Acne moderate

Localized nodules. They can be painful, hard to heal or both, with small wounds.

Chapter 11: How Does Posture Affect Testosterone?

We know that a the correct posture and testosterone levels affect the health of a person. The way you speak can have profound impacts on stress levels as well as hormones.

Poses with confidence that are different from the closed posture, and that require less pressure can raise testosterone levels by as much as 20%, and decrease the levels of cortisol by 25 percent in just 2 minutes.

Now, dear friends, stand straight and draw your shoulders to the side.

Treatments for male hypogonadism

Doctors will determine if the condition is male hypogonadism. This can be determined through an examination of your body as well as test of your blood. If your physician detects lower testosterone levels, they can run additional tests in order to pinpoint the root cause.

The treatment usually includes TRT, or testosterone treatment (TRT) as a type of

Gels

Patches

Injections

The treatment of replacement for testosterone (TRT) is believed to aid in

Muscle mass reduce

The energy sector is boosted

Restorative treatment for sexual function

Treatment for Testosterone Replacement Therapy (TRT) for men who are healthy ?

There are many people who experience changes in their age similar to signs of hypogonadism. However, their symptoms might not be due to any type of disease or accident. They are often viewed as an ordinary aspect of aging for instance.

A normal part of aging, there are many who experience symptoms is similar to symptoms that are common in hypogonadism, but the symptoms might not be related to a illness or accident.

Self-confidence

A decrease in motivation

Muscles are less

Increased body fat

Sexual role

Sleep patterns are changing

TRT may help those suffering from hypogonadism. Results are less favorable for people who have normal testosterone levels, or those with a lower levels of testosterone.

The recommendation for Hormone Supplements

A decrease in testosterone levels could result in unpleasant and uncomfortable signs and symptoms. Our opinions is a bit skewed on how serious low levels of testosterone should be considered and the best way to be handled.

A low testosterone level can lead to horrifying and debilitating symptoms. However, opinions differ about whether or not testosterone levels should be decreased.

The potential risks of testosterone supplements are

www.ingramcontent.com/pod-product-compliance
Lightning Source LLC
Chambersburg PA
CBHW060224030426
42335CB00014B/1329